PEARSON

EKG Technician Program
Advanced

Second Custom Edition for Condensed Curriculum International

Taken from:
EKG: Plain and Simple, Fourth Edition
by Karen M. Ellis, RN

Cover Art: TK

Taken from:

EKG: Plain and Simple, Fourth Edition
by Karen M. Ellis, RN
Copyright © 2017, 2012, 2007 by Pearson Education, Inc.
New York, NY 10013

This special edition published in cooperation with Pearson Education, Inc.

Pearson Education, Inc., 330 Hudson Street, New York, New York 10013
A Pearson Education Company
www.pearsoned.com

Printed in the United States of America

000200010272102029

NH

PEARSON   ISBN 10: 1-323-74614-5
ISBN 13: 978-1-323-74614-1

Contents

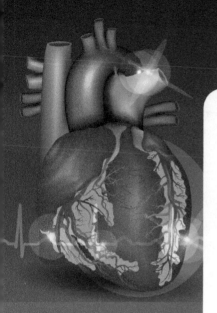

How to Interpret a 12-Lead EKG

CHAPTER 1 OBJECTIVES

Upon completion of this chapter, the student will be able to

- Differentiate normal versus abnormal QRS configurations on the 12-lead EKG.
- List the six steps to 12-lead EKG interpretation.
- Determine the axis quadrant on a variety of practice EKGs.
- Determine if right or left bundle branch blocks exist.
- Determine the presence of left anterior and left posterior hemiblocks.
- Identify right and left ventricular hypertrophy.
- Determine if any miscellaneous effects are present.

What It's All About

Mr. Seybourne has a history of kidney failure and has been told he will soon need dialysis. "I'm trying to hold off as long as I can," Mr. Seybourne tells his nurse as she does an EKG and draws blood for lab work. The nurse notes markedly tall pointy T waves on the EKG, consistent with hyperkalemia. She alerts the physician, who tells Mr. Seybourne that based on the EKG it looks like his potassium level is very high and he may need to start dialysis tonight. "You can tell how my labs are going to look just by looking at my EKG?" Mr. Seybourne asks the physician. "Yes, the EKG can tell us a lot of information about other things besides the heart," the physician answers. Soon the lab results are back and the potassium level is indeed alarmingly high. Other labs are also markedly elevated, so the physician advises Mr. Seybourne that he can't hold off any longer—he must start his dialysis emergently tonight.

Introduction

The 12-lead EKG is a diagnostic test done primarily to identify the presence of myocardial infarction or ischemia, but it is also useful in identifying arrhythmias, electrolyte imbalances, drug toxicities, and other conditions. It is done with the patient at rest, usually in the supine (back-lying) position. As with rhythm interpretation, it is important to use a systematic method of assessment.

The Six Steps to 12-Lead EKG Interpretation

Use these steps in order:

1. *Interpret the basics—Identify the rhythm and calculate heart rate and intervals (PR, QRS, QT).* These were covered in Part I of the text. If the EKG has a rhythm strip at the bottom, assess the basics here. Otherwise, pick any lead (Leads II and V_1 are the best ones to evaluate for rhythm). Do the intervals fall within normal limits or are they abnormally shortened or prolonged? Prolonged PR intervals can imply a block in conduction between the atria and ventricles,

whereas shortened PR intervals can signal a change in the heart's pacemaker. Prolonged QRS intervals can imply a ventricular rhythm, a block of one of the bundle branches, or electrolyte (blood chemical) abnormalities. Prolonged QT intervals can herald the potential for lethal arrhythmias and can imply medication side effects.

2. *Determine the axis quadrant.*   Is it normal or is there axis deviation? Axis is simply a method of determining the mean direction of current flow in the heart.

3. *Check for bundle branch blocks and hemiblocks (a block of a branch of the left bundle branch).*

4. *Check for ventricular hypertrophy (overgrowth of myocardial tissue).*   Use V_1 and V_{5-6} to check the QRS complexes for signs of ventricular hypertrophy.

5. *Determine the presence of miscellaneous effects.*   Examine all leads for disturbances in calcium or potassium levels in the bloodstream and for digitalis effects.

6. *Check for myocardial infarction/ischemia.*   For this you'll look at all leads except aVR. You'll look for ST elevation or depression, inverted T waves, and significant Q waves. You'll also note R wave progression in the precordial leads. This will be covered in depth in Chapter 2.

Before we get started, let's recall the normal QRS configuration on the 12 lead EKG.

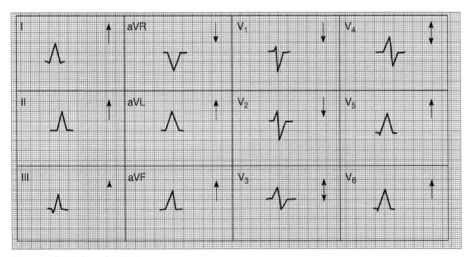

Normal 12-lead EKG.
The arrows indicate the correct deflection of the QRS complexes.

Now let's practice identifying normal versus abnormal QRS configurations.

Lead Morphology Practice

Determine if the following QRS morphologies are normal. If not, tell what the abnormality is.

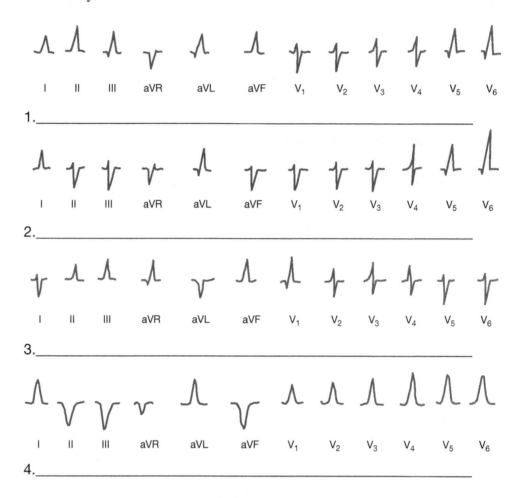

1._____

2._____

3._____

4._____

Just by analyzing the morphology of each lead, we can get an idea of whether there is any pathology on the EKG. Three of the preceding four EKGs were abnormal in some way. As we continue further along, we will learn the implications of this abnormality, and we'll learn more ways to analyze EKGs. Let's move on to axis quadrant determination.

Axis Quadrant Determination

The electrical axis is a method of depicting the direction of the heart's electrical current flow. Recall that the heart's current starts normally in the sinus node and travels downward toward the left ventricle. If we drew an arrow depicting this current flow, it would point downward to the left. In abnormal hearts or abnormal rhythms, this current may travel in an unusual direction, resulting in an axis deviation (the arrow would point in a different direction).

Causes of Axis Deviations

- *Normal variant.* It may be normal for some individuals to have an abnormal axis. Keep in mind that "abnormal" does not necessarily mean pathological. As physicians often say, "That's normal for *you*."
- *Myocardial infarction.* Infarcted (dead) tissue does not conduct electrical current, so the current detours around and away from this dead tissue, shifting the axis away.

- *Ventricular hypertrophy.* Hypertrophied (overgrown) tissue requires more current to depolarize it, so the current shifts toward the hypertrophied area.
- *Arrhythmias.* Arrhythmias can cause axis deviation. Ventricular rhythms, for example, start in the ventricle and send their current upward toward the atria. The axis would then point upward rather than downward.
- *Advanced pregnancy or obesity.* These conditions physically push the diaphragm and the heart upward, causing the axis to shift upward to the left.
- *Chronic lung disease and pulmonary embolism.* These conditions cause a rightward axis shift because they enlarge the right ventricle.
- *Hemiblocks.* These blocks of one of the branches of the left bundle branch cause impulses to travel in an alternate direction, resulting in either a right axis deviation or a left axis deviation.

Determining the Axis Quadrant

Because the axis is concerned with direction, axis calculation requires a compass. A compass has lines delineating north, south, east, and west. In axis calculation, our compass is the hexiaxial diagram superimposed on the heart, as seen in Figure 1–1. The hexiaxial diagram has lines depicting the frontal leads—I, II, III, aVR, aVL, and aVF. Lead I runs right to left, and aVF runs up and down. The other leads are points in between. The leads are separated from one another by 30° increments. The axis circle is made by joining the ends of these lead lines. Note the degree markings in Figure 1–1. The current of the heart flowing from the sinus node to the left ventricle would yield an axis of about 60°. That is a normal axis.

If we use Leads I and aVF to divide the axis circle into four quadrants, normal axis would be between 0 and +90°. Left axis deviation is between 0 and −90°. Right axis deviation is between +90 and ± 180°. Indeterminate axis (so-called because it cannot be determined whether it is an extreme left axis deviation or an extreme right axis deviation) is between −90 and ± 180°. Note the axis quadrants in Figure 1–1.

Look at the QRS in Leads I and aVF to determine the axis quadrant. Because Lead I connects right and left arms, it tells us whether the heart's current is traveling to the right or left; aVF is located on the leg, so it tells us whether the heart's current is traveling upward or downward. If the QRS in both Leads I and aVF is positive, the axis is normal. If the QRS in Lead I is positive and the one in aVF is negative, it is left axis deviation (LAD). If Lead I and aVF are both negative, it is indeterminate axis. If Lead I is negative but aVF is positive, it is right axis deviation (RAD). See Figure 1–2.

> **QuickTip**
>
> If Leads I and aVF are both upright, you could say they're "two thumbs up" and that's always good (normal).

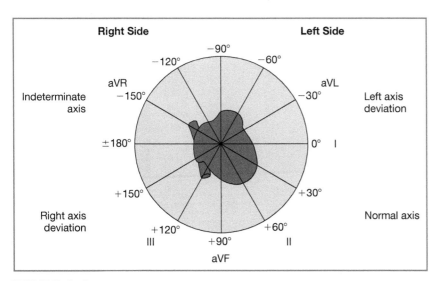

FIGURE 1–1

Axis circle and quadrants.

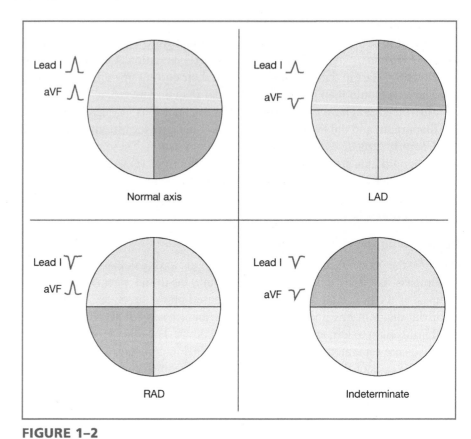

FIGURE 1–2

Determining the axis quadrant.

It is important to compare the axis on the current EKG with the previous EKG. If the axis has changed, look for conditions that may be responsible. Did the patient have an MI? Is there an arrhythmia? Is the patient in advanced pregnancy or has she recently delivered? Has the patient's pulmonary disease worsened? Is there a pulmonary embolus (blood clot in the lung)? The axis is a clue. Use it to help find the problem.

Axis Practice EKGs

Determine the axis quadrant on the following EKGs.

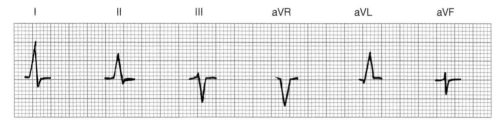

1. Axis quadrant = _____

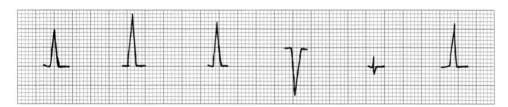

2. Axis quadrant = _____

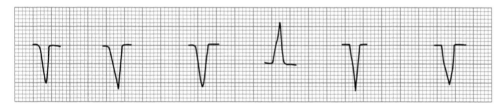

3. Axis quadrant = _____

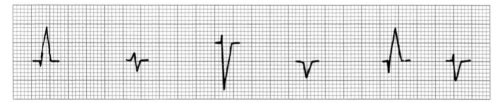

4. Axis quadrant = _____

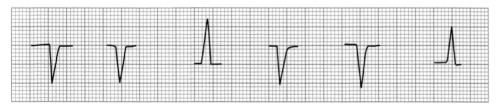

5. Axis quadrant = _____

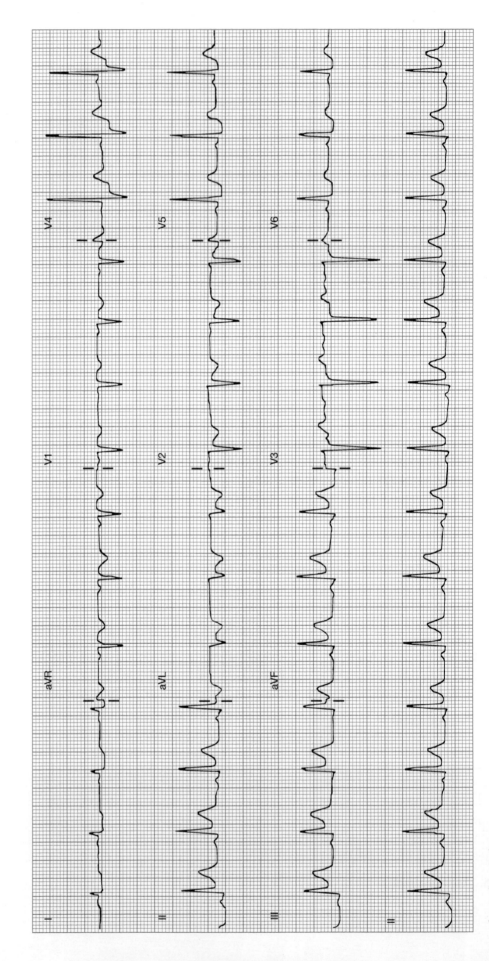

8

6. Axis quadrant = _____

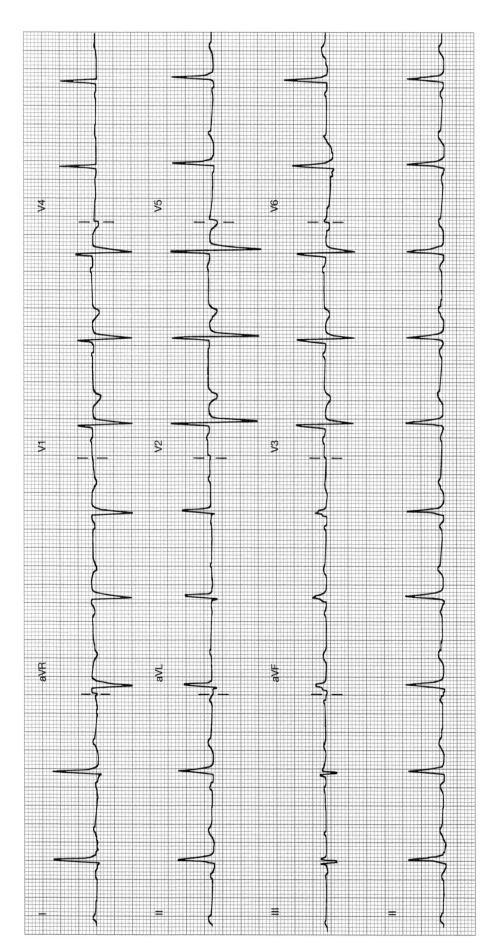

7. Axis quadrant = _____

Bundle Branch Blocks

Bundle branch blocks occur when either the right or left bundle branch becomes blocked and unable to conduct impulses, often as a result of heart disease. The electrical impulse travels rapidly down the healthy bundle branch and then must trudge very slowly, cell by cell, through the affected ventricle. This difference in impulse conduction in the two ventricles causes the ventricles to depolarize consecutively instead of simultaneously, causing a widened QRS complex with a characteristic QRS configuration. *Bundle branch blocks are seen only in supraventricular (sinus, atrial, or junctional) rhythms,* because only these rhythms require conduction through the bundle branches. Ventricular rhythms are formed in the ventricular tissue below the bundle branch system and do not use the bundle branches for impulse conduction. Therefore, *ventricular rhythms cannot exhibit bundle branch blocks.*

In Figure 1–3, note the normal anatomy of the bundle branch system. The right bundle branch is located on the right side of the interventricular septum. The left bundle branch is on the left side of the septum. You'll note the left bundle branch has two divisions called fascicles. Fascicles are branches. In order to understand the QRS complexes produced by bundle branch blocks, let's first review normal conduction through the bundle branch system. We'll look at Lead V_1 because this lead is the best for interpreting bundle branch blocks. See Figure 1–4. You'll recall that the heart's normal current starts in the sinus node and travels toward the left ventricle—top to bottom, right to left. Because V_1's electrode sits to the right of the heart, it sees a little current traveling toward it (across the septum toward the right ventricle), then the bulk of the current traveling away from it toward the left ventricle. You'll recall that an impulse traveling away from a positive electrode writes a negative deflection. V_1's QRS complex is, therefore, primarily negative, showing a small R wave and then a deeper S wave.

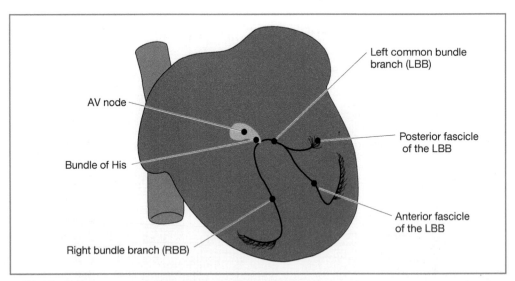

FIGURE 1–3

Bundle branch system anatomy.

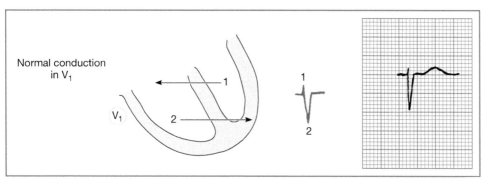

FIGURE 1–4

Normal conduction in V₁: (1) septal and beginning right ventricular activation, (2) left ventricular activation.

Right Bundle Branch Block (RBBB)

See Figure 1–5. In *right bundle branch block* (RBBB), the QRS complex typically starts out looking normal—primarily negative—indicating initial normal travel through the heart via the healthy left bundle branch. But then the QRS has an extra R wave at the end, signifying the current that's slogging slowly, cell by cell, through the right ventricle toward V₁'s electrode. Thus, V₁ has an R wave, an S wave, then another R wave. This second R wave is called **R prime** and is written R′. Occasionally a RBBB will lose its initial R wave and will instead have a small Q wave and then a prominent R wave.

All bundle branch blocks will have a QRS interval of ≥0.12 seconds and a T wave that slopes off opposite the terminal wave of the QRS complex. If the terminal wave of the QRS is upward, for example, the T wave will be inverted. If the terminal wave of the QRS is downward, the T wave will be upright. See Figure 1–5. In V₁, the QRS interval is 0.14 secs and the terminal wave of the QRS is upright, so the T wave is inverted. It is important to recognize these bundle-related T waves so as not to misinterpret them as signs of ischemia. See Figure 1–6 for a RBBB on a 12-lead EKG.

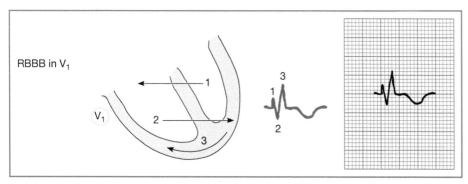

FIGURE 1–5

RBBB in V₁: (1) septal and beginning right ventricular activation, (2) left ventricular activation, (3) final right ventricular activation.

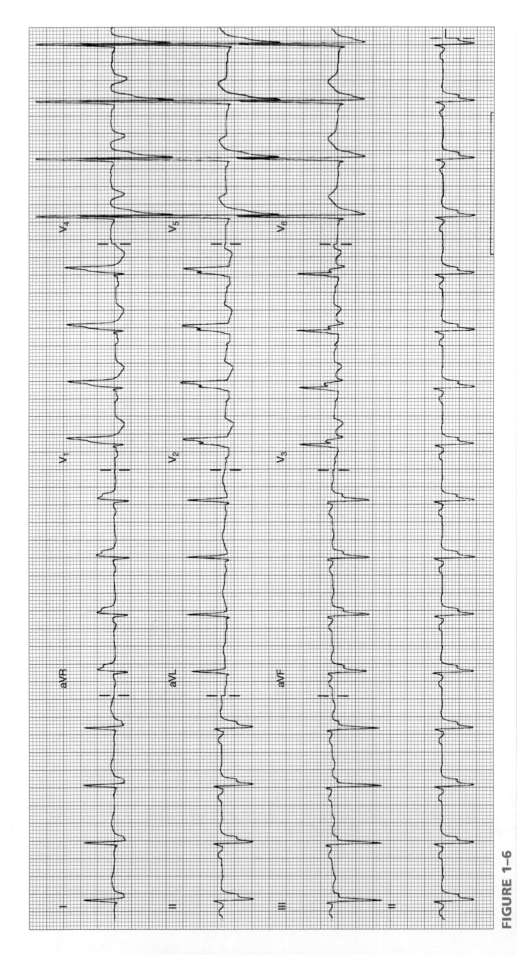

FIGURE 1-6

Right bundle branch block. Note the RSR′ in V$_1$ along with the QRS interval ≥0.12 seconds and the T waves opposite the terminal QRS wave.

Left Bundle Branch Block (LBBB)

Left bundle branch block (LBBB) can occur in two ways: There can be a block of the left common bundle branch (the part of the left bundle branch before it divides into its fascicles) or a block of both fascicles. In either case, depolarization of the septum cannot occur normally in LBBB. See Figure 1–7. Septal depolarization must go backward, right to left, sending its current away from V_1's positive electrode. When the current reaches the left ventricle, it finds the bundle branch blocked and must traverse the left ventricular tissue slowly, one cell at a time. Meanwhile, right ventricular activation is occurring normally through the healthy right bundle branch. In Figure 1–7, numbers 1 and 2 are invisible inside number 3, as the huge amount of current required to activate the left ventricle dwarfs the current traveling to the septum and right ventricle. The slowed travel through the left ventricle results in a wider-than-normal S wave. LBBB in V_1 thus presents as a large, deep QS complex in V_1. On occasion, there may be a small R wave preceding the deep S wave. As with a RBBB, the QRS interval of a LBBB will be ≥0.12 secs, and the T wave will be opposite the terminal wave of the QRS complex. See Figure 1–8 for a LBBB on a 12-lead EKG. See Figure 1–9 for a summary of the criteria for bundle branch blocks.

Rate-Related BBB

Bundle branch blocks seen only at certain heart rates are known as rate-related bundle branch blocks, and the rate at which the BBB appears is called the critical rate. In this disorder, conduction through the bundle branches is normal at heart rates below the critical rate. Once the critical rate is reached, however, one of the bundle branches becomes incapable of depolarizing rapidly enough to allow normal conduction, and a BBB results. When the heart rate falls below the critical rate, bundle branch depolarization returns to normal and the BBB disappears.

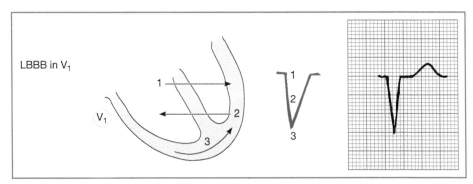

FIGURE 1–7

LBBB in V_1: (1) septal and beginning left ventricular activation, (2) right ventricular activation, (3) final left ventricular activation.

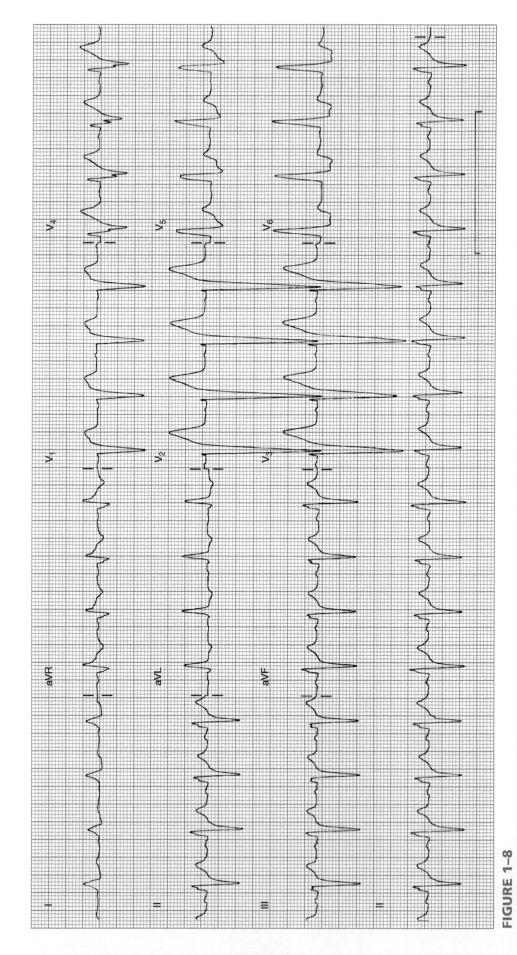

FIGURE 1–8

Left bundle branch block. Note the RS configuration in V_1 along with the widened QRS interval (≥0.12 seconds) and the T wave opposite the terminal wave of the QRS.

Type of BBB	QRS configuration in V_1	QRS interval	T wave	Causes
RBBB	RSR' 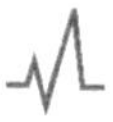	≥0.12 secs	Opposite the terminal QRS	• Coronary artery disease • Conduction system lesion • Normal variant • Right ventricular hypertrophy • Congenital heart disease • Right ventricular dilatation
LBBB	QS or RS 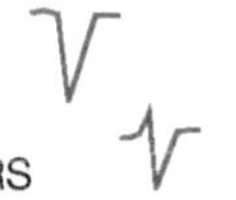	≥0.12 secs	Opposite the terminal QRS	• Coronary artery disease • Conduction system lesion • Hypertension • Other organic heart disease

FIGURE 1–9

Summary of criteria for bundle branch blocks.

Clinical Implications of BBB

Bundle branch blocks do not typically cause symptoms. In fact, they *are* a symptom of an impaired conduction system. The question is what's causing the BBB? See Table 1–1. Although RBBB can be seen in normal healthy hearts, LBBB almost always implies cardiac disease. Patients with bundle branch block are at risk for developing severe AV blocks (e.g., if both bundle branches become blocked simultaneously), so it is important to observe their rhythm closely for further signs of conduction disturbance, such as a new first-degree AV block. *A new bundle branch block should prompt an immediate assessment of the patient.* A 12-lead EKG should be done in an effort to determine the cause of the BBB. Remember—*the BBB is a symptom of another problem.* For example, the BBB might be a result of an MI in progress. Also remember that BBBs cause T wave changes that can be misinterpreted as ischemia. Certain kinds of MIs can be difficult to diagnose in the presence of an LBBB, as the bundle-related changes mask the MI.

TABLE 1–1   Causes of RBBB and LBBB

Type of BBB	Causes
RBBB	• Coronary artery disease • Conduction system lesion • Normal variant • Right ventricular hypertrophy • Congenital heart disease • Right ventricular dilatation
LBBB	• Coronary artery disease • Conduction system lesion • Hypertension • Other organic heart disease

chapter CHECKUP

We're about halfway through this chapter. To evaluate your understanding of the material thus far, answer the following questions. If you have trouble with them, review the material again before continuing.

1. Name the steps for EKG interpretation.
2. State the causes of axis deviation.
3. Determine the axis quadrant if the QRS is positive in Leads I and aVF, and if both are negative.
4. State the criteria for RBBB and LBBB.

Hemiblock

A *hemiblock* is a block of one of the fascicles of the left bundle branch. There are two kinds of hemiblocks: left anterior hemiblock (LAHB), a block in the left anterior fascicle of the left bundle branch, and left posterior hemiblock (LPHB), a block in the posterior fascicle.

Unlike bundle branch blocks, hemiblocks do not cause QRS widening, but they do cause axis deviation. Left anterior hemiblock results in left axis deviation, and left posterior hemiblock results in right axis deviation. LAHB is much more common than LPHB because LPHB has a dual blood supply—the circumflex and right coronary arteries—and LAHB has only a single blood supply—the left anterior descending coronary artery. Hemiblocks that occur alone are not usually clinically significant. If they occur simultaneously with RBBB, however—a condition called a bifascicular block—this development can predispose the patient to AV blocks because two of the conduction pathways to the ventricle are now blocked. Hemiblocks are caused by the same factors that cause bundle branch blocks. Treatment is not required for hemiblocks per se, but treat AV blocks if they occur. See Figure 1–10 for hemiblock configurations.

Now let's look at an algorithm for bundle branch blocks and hemiblocks. You can use Figure 1–11 to help decide if there's a BBB and/or hemiblock, and what kind it is. Look back at Figure 1–6. We know there's a RBBB there but there's also a hemiblock. Can you tell what kind?

It's LAHB. See the left axis deviation along with the RBBB?

Now let's practice. Look for BBBs and hemiblocks.

QuickTip

Hemiblocks can accompany right bundle branch blocks but not left bundle branch blocks. LBBB already implies that both fascicles are blocked.

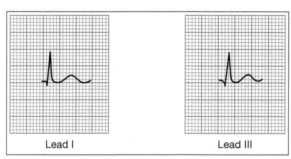

Normal QRS configuration in leads I and III.

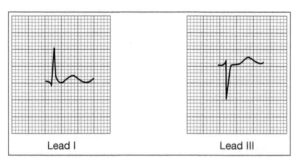

QRS configuration in LAHB.

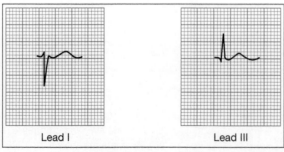

QRS configuration in LPHB.

FIGURE 1–10

QRS configuration in hemiblocks.

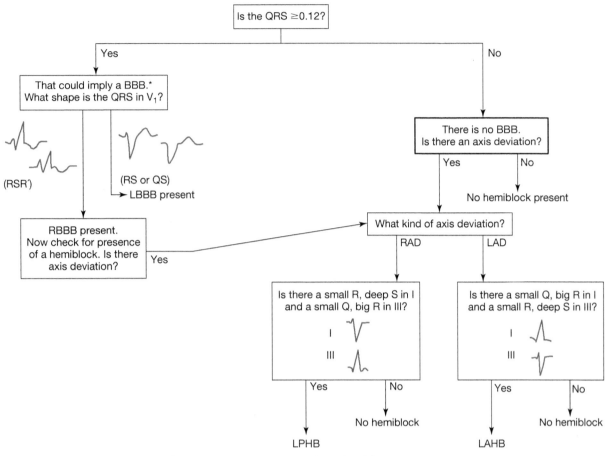

*Wide QRS complexes could be ventricular in origin, rather than a BBB.

FIGURE 1–11

Bundle branch block/hemiblock algorithm.

BBB Practice

1. Type of BBB/HB (if any): _____

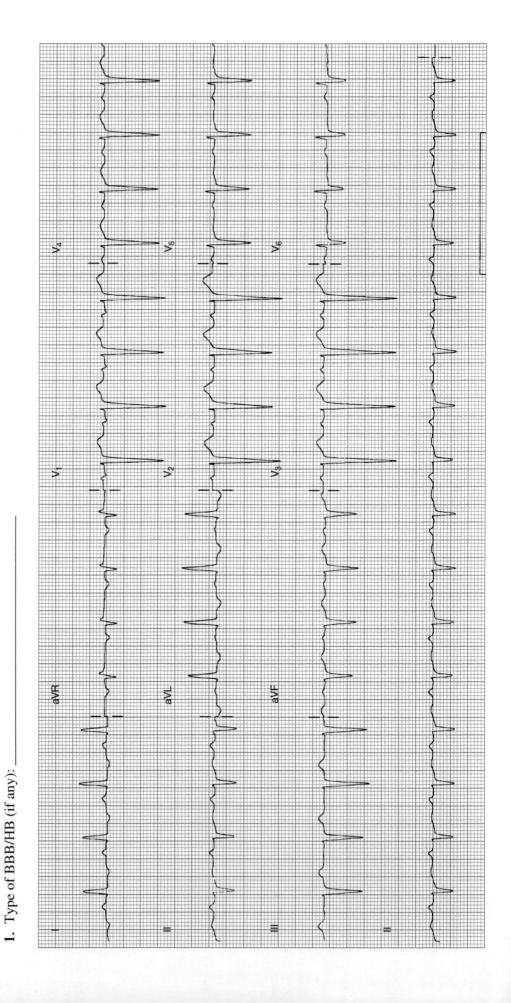

2. Type of BBB/HB (if any): _____

3. Type of BBB/HB (if any): _____

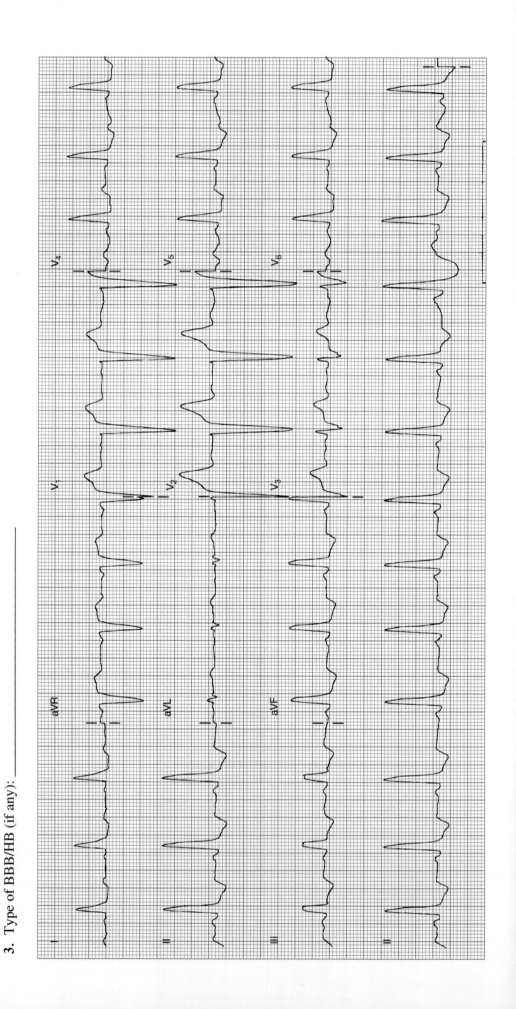

4. Type of BBB/HB (if any): _____

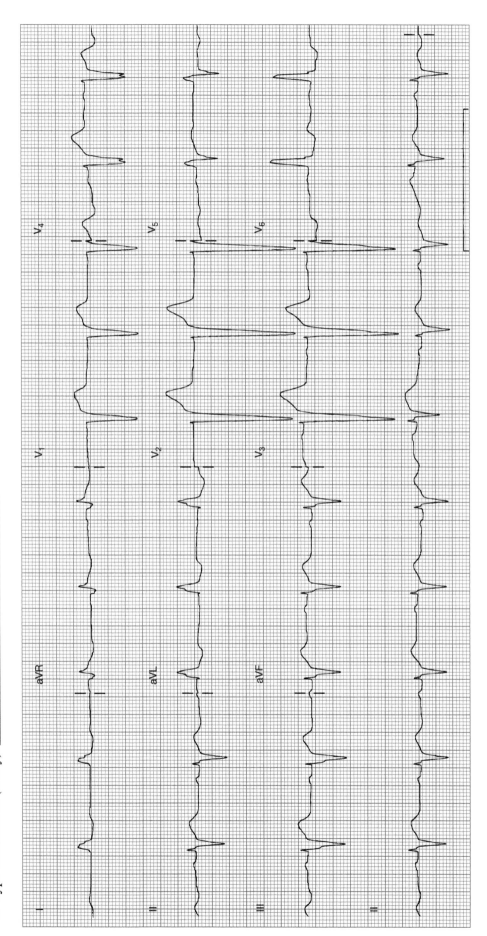

5. Type of BBB/HB (if any): _____

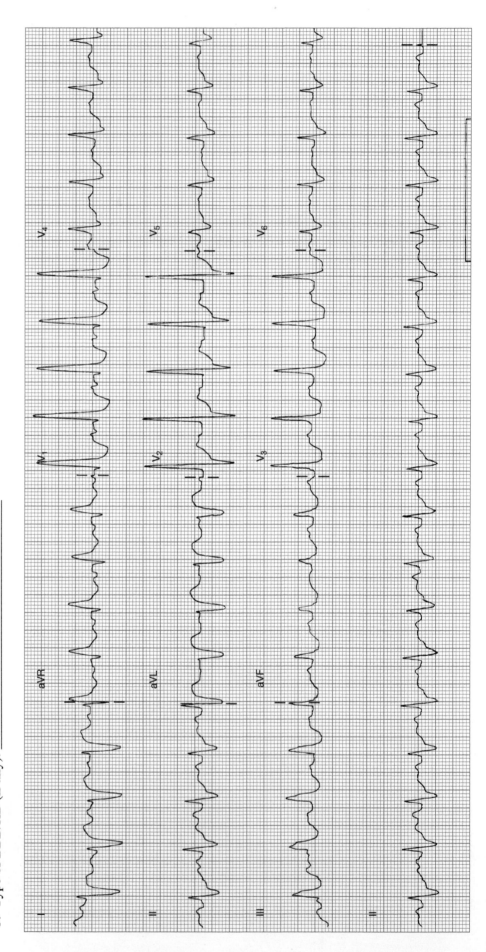

6. Type of BBB/HB (if any): _____

7. Type of BBB/HB (if any): _____

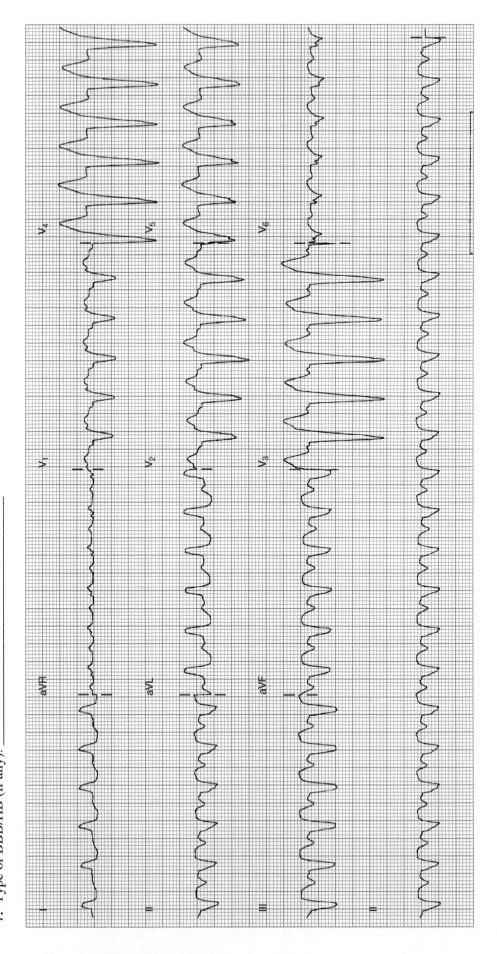

8. Type of BBB/HB (if any): _____

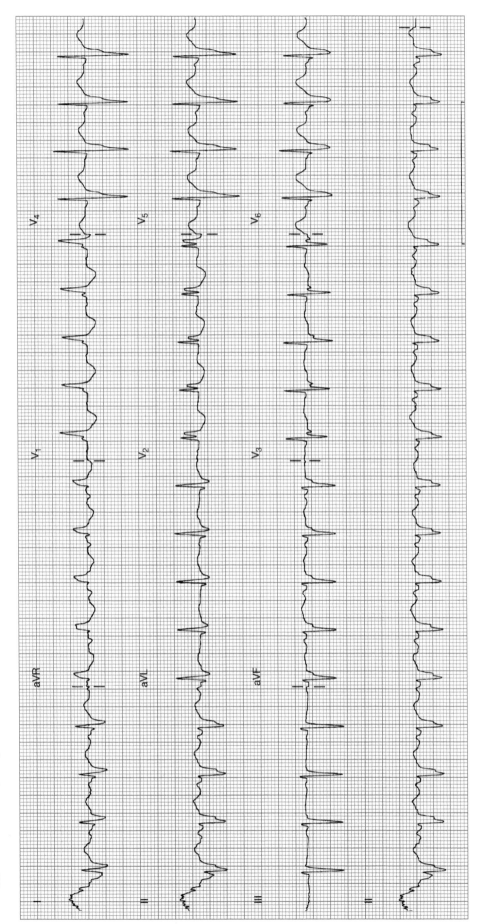

9. Type of BBB/HB (if any): _____

10. Type of BBB/HB (if any): _____

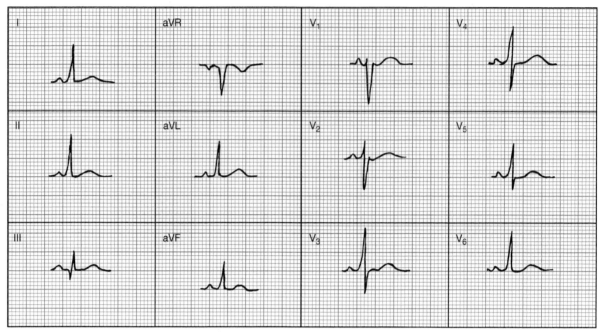

FIGURE 1–12

Normal QRS amplitude (voltage).

Ventricular Hypertrophy

Hypertrophy refers to excessive growth of tissue. In ventricular hypertrophy, the muscle mass of the right or left ventricle (or both) is thickened, usually as a result of disease. This thickened tissue requires more current to depolarize it and thus causes greater-than-normal amplitude of the QRS complexes in the leads over the hypertrophied ventricle. Let's look at an example of normal QRS amplitude. See Figure 1–12. *The normal QRS complex should be no taller or deeper than 13 mm high (13 small blocks) in any lead.*

Right Ventricular Hypertrophy (RVH)

Right ventricular hypertrophy (RVH) is evidenced on the EKG by a tall R wave in V_1 (greater than or equal to the size of the S wave), accompanied by a right axis deviation and, often noted but not required, T wave inversion. The R wave in V_1 represents depolarization of the right ventricle, so it will be taller than normal if the right ventricle is enlarged. The most common cause of RVH is chronic lung disease, which forces the right ventricle to bulk up in order to force its blood out into the now high-pressure lung system. See Figure 1–13 for an example of the typical QRST configuration in RVH in V_1.

Now let's see what RVH looks like on a 12-lead EKG. See Figure 1–14.

Left Ventricular Hypertrophy (LVH)

Left ventricular hypertrophy (LVH) is most commonly caused by hypertension (high blood pressure), which causes the left ventricle to bulk up in order to expel its blood against the great resistance of the abnormally high blood pressure.

LVH has several possible criteria but the one most commonly used is the following:

R wave in V_5 or V_6 (whichever is taller) + the S wave in V_1 or V_2 ≥ 35 mm

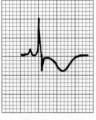

FIGURE 1–13

QRST configuration typical of RVH in V_1.

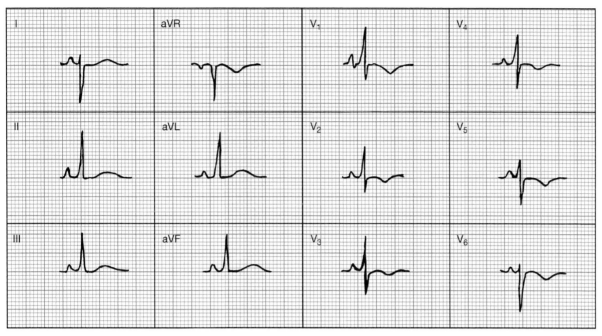

FIGURE 1–14

Right ventricular hypertrophy. Note that the R wave in V₁ is taller than the S wave is deep; there is right axis deviation and T wave inversion.

In LVH, Leads I, aVL, V₅, and V₆ will have taller-than-normal R waves as the current travels toward their positive electrodes; Leads V₁ and V₂ will have deeper-than-normal S waves as the current travels away from their positive electrode. See Figure 1–15. Add the height of the R wave in V₅ to the depth of the S wave in V₁. The result is ≥35 mm. This is LVH by voltage criteria. See Figure 1–16 for a 12-lead EKG example of LVH.

Ventricular hypertrophy does not usually prolong the QRS interval beyond normal limits.

Low-Voltage EKGs

Some people have abnormally low-voltage EKGs, in which the waves and complexes are shorter than usual. See Figure 1–17. Note the difference in voltage between this EKG and the normal one in Figure 1–12. Low-voltage EKGs, contrary to what may seem logical, do not imply that the heart is smaller than normal, or that it is generating less current than normal. It is usually caused by an outside influence that affects the heart's current on its way to the electrodes on the skin.

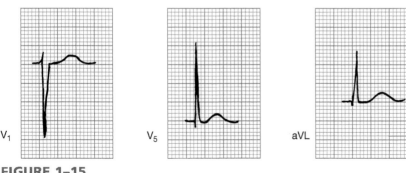

FIGURE 1–15

LVH by voltage criteria.

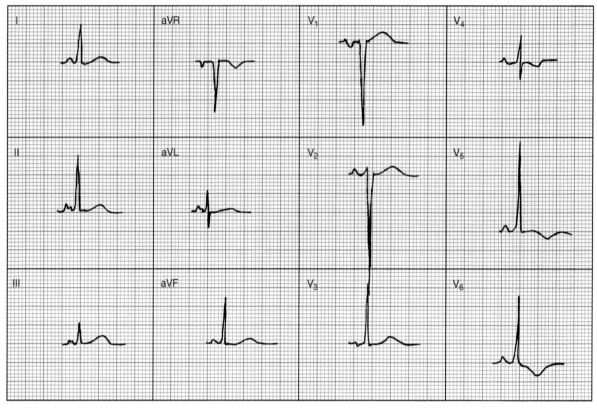

FIGURE 1–16

Left ventricular hypertrophy. Note the S wave in V_1 is 22 mm deep, and the R in V_5 is 24 mm tall, for a total voltage of 46 mm. This meets and exceeds the criteria for LVH.

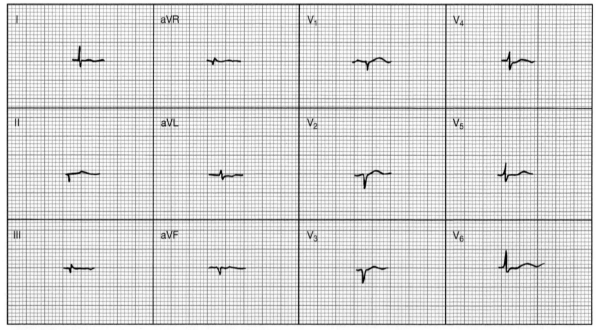

FIGURE 1–17

Low-voltage EKG.

The following are some possible causes of a low-voltage EKG:

- *Obesity.*   Fatty tissue muffles the cardiac impulse on its way to the electrodes on the skin.
- *Emphysema.*   Air trapping in the lungs muffles the impulse.
- *Myxedema.*   The thyroid gland function is abnormally low, causing decreased voltage.
- *Pericardial effusion.*   Excessive fluid inside the pericardial sac surrounding the heart muffles the impulse on its way to the skin.

Clinical Implications of Hypertrophy

Hypertrophy is the heart's way of attempting to meet a contractile demand that cannot be met by normal-size heart muscle. Unfortunately, hypertrophy also places increased demands on the coronary circulation to feed that extra muscle bulk. When that increased blood and oxygen demand cannot be adequately met, ischemia results. Hypertrophy increases the likelihood of ischemia and infarction simply by increasing the amount of muscle mass to be nourished by the coronary arteries.

Ventricular dilatation, a stretching of the myocardial fibers that results from overfilling of the ventricles or inadequate pumping of blood out of the ventricles, can also result in a hypertrophy pattern on the EKG.

Hypertrophy Practice

Look for hypertrophy and low voltage on the following EKGs. Your answer will be one of these: RVH, LVH, low voltage, or normal.

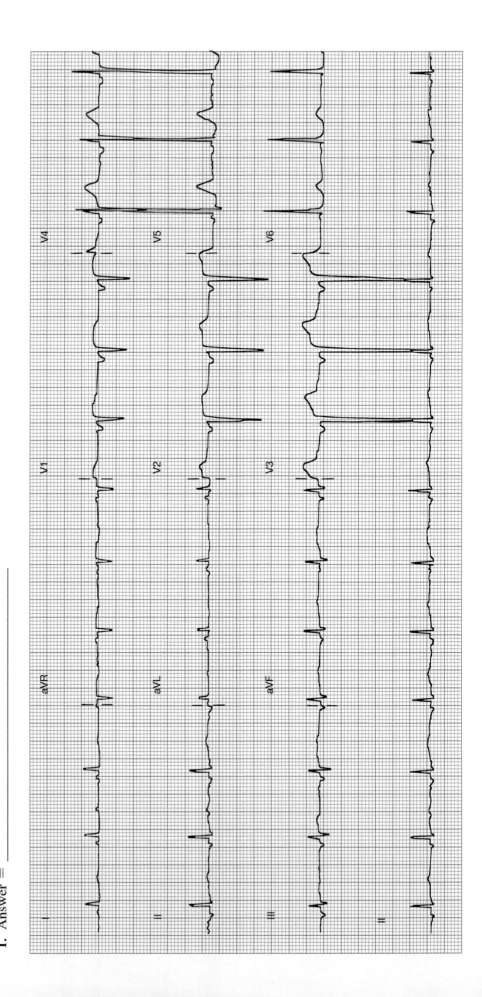

1. Answer = _____

2. Answer = _____

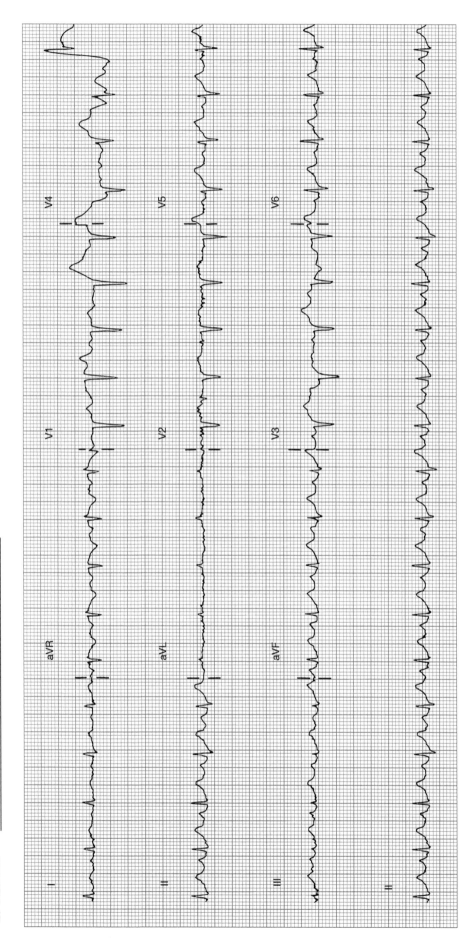

33

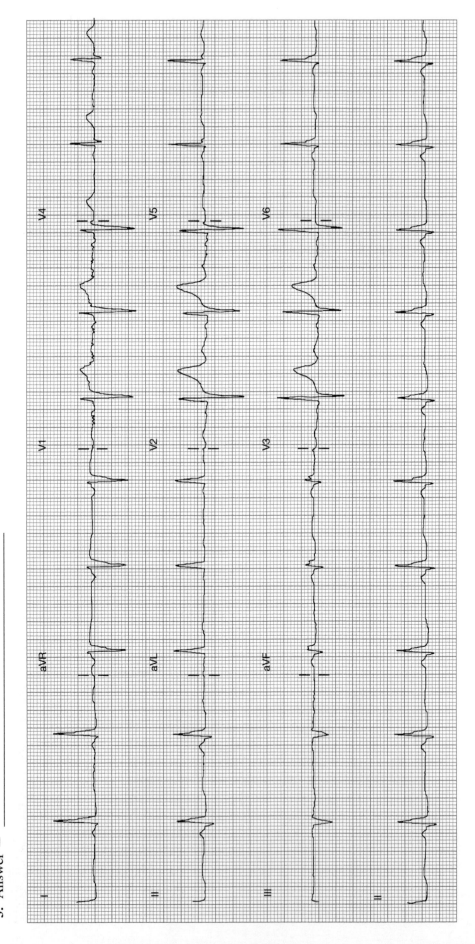

3. Answer = _____

4. Answer = _____

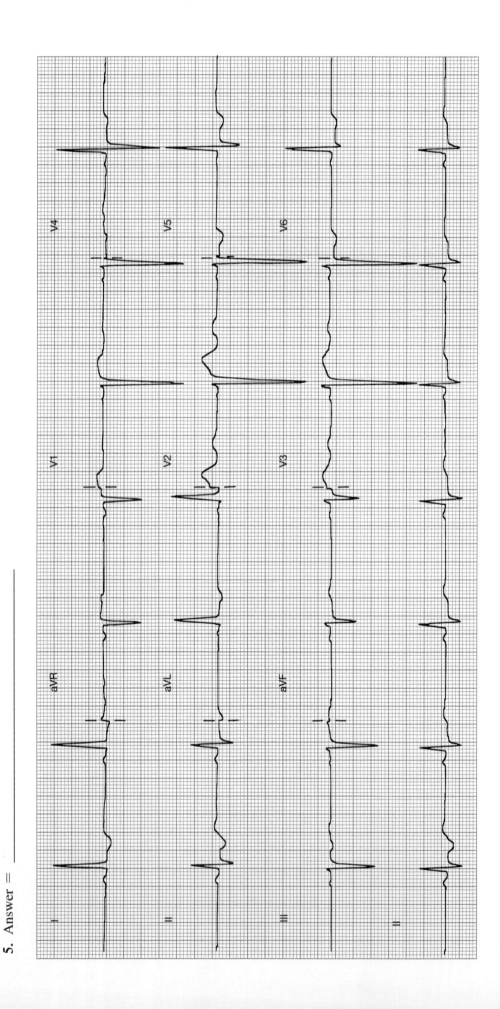

5. Answer = _____

Miscellaneous Effects

Electrolyte (blood chemicals) abnormalities and certain medications can affect the EKG. Let's look at some of these effects.

Digitalis Effect

Digitalis is a medication given to increase the force of myocardial contraction in patients with heart failure, or to slow the heart rate in patients with tachycardias. Digitalis medications are notorious for causing sagging ST segment depression (also called a *scooping* ST segment) that is easily misinterpreted as ischemia. The cause of this ST segment change is still not understood. Digitalis slows conduction through the AV node, potentially resulting in a prolonged PR interval. These effects are not necessarily indicative of digitalis toxicity (excessive digitalis in the bloodstream), as they also occur at normal therapeutic levels. See Figure 1–18. See the sagging, very rounded ST segments and prolonged PR interval? This is typical of the digitalis effect.

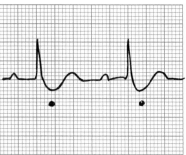

FIGURE 1–18

Digitalis effect.

Electrolyte Abnormalities

Hyperkalemia

Hyperkalemia, a high potassium level in the bloodstream, has two main EKG effects. First, potassium levels of about 6 cause tall, pointy, narrow T waves. (Normal blood potassium level is around 3.5 to 5.) As the potassium level rises to around 8, the tall T wave may be replaced by a widened QRS complex. This widened QRS is a sign that cardiac arrest may be imminent if the potassium level is not lowered quickly. These EKG effects are due to potassium's effect on depolarization and repolarization and will return to normal once the potassium level is normalized. One way to remember potassium's effect on the T wave is to think of the T wave as a tent containing potassium: the more potassium, the taller the tent. See Figure 1–19. In Figure 1–19A, note the tall, pointy T waves. In Figure 1–19B, note the widened QRS complex.

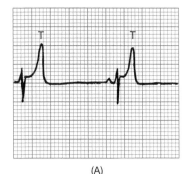

(A)

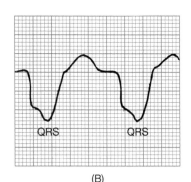

(B)

FIGURE 1–19

Hyperkalemia.

Hypokalemia

A low potassium level in the bloodstream results in a prominent U wave and flattened T waves. The potassium tent is almost empty, so it flattens out. These effects occur because repolarization, especially phase 3 of the action potential, is disturbed by the potassium deficit. See Figure 1–20.

Note the flattened T wave and the prominent U wave in Figure 1–20. Recall the U wave is not usually seen on the EKG, but if it is present it follows the T wave. T waves always follow QRS complexes. *If there are no obvious T waves on the strip, be sure the QRS complexes are really QRS complexes and not artifact.* Then, if you still can't see T waves following those QRS complexes, you can be reasonably sure the potassium level is quite low, usually around a blood level of 2.0. T waves will improve after supplemental potassium is given.

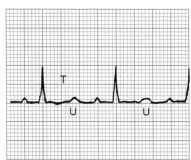

FIGURE 1–20

Hypokalemia.

Hypercalcemia

Hypercalcemia, an elevated blood calcium level, causes the ST segment to shorten to such an extent that the T wave seems to be almost on top of the QRS. This effect occurs because the elevated calcium level shortens the repolarization phase of the action potential. See Figure 1–21.

In Figure 1–21, note the extremely short ST segment that results in a short QT interval. The ST segment and QT interval will return to normal once the calcium level is normalized.

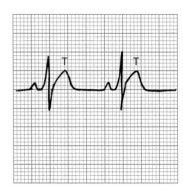

FIGURE 1–21

Hypercalcemia.

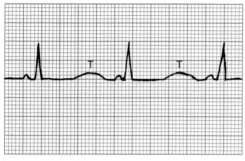

FIGURE 1–22

Hypocalcemia.

Hypocalcemia

Hypocalcemia, low calcium level in the bloodstream, prolongs repolarization and causes a prolonged ST segment, thus prolonging the QT interval.

In Figure 1–22, note how far the T wave is from the QRS complex. This demonstrates a very prolonged ST segment and QT interval.

See Figure 1–23 for a summary of miscellaneous effects.

We now can evaluate *almost all* of a 12-lead EKG with one very important exception—we need to know if our patient is having an MI. Let's check that out in the next chapter.

EFFECT	EKG CHANGE
Digitalis effect	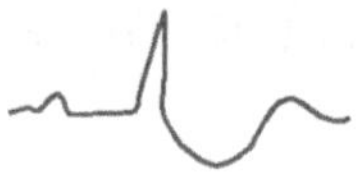 Prolonged PR interval, sagging ST segment depression
Hyperkalemia	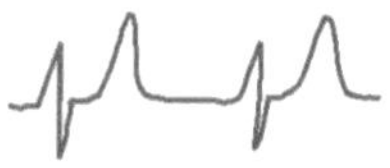 Tall, narrow, pointy T waves
Severe hyperkalemia	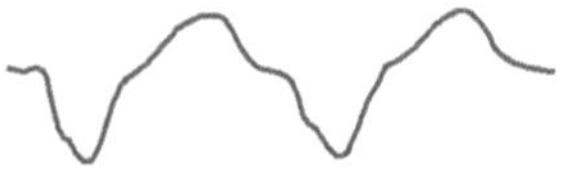 Widened QRS complex
Hypokalemia	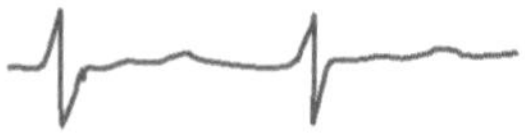 Flattened T wave, prominent U wave
Hypercalcemia	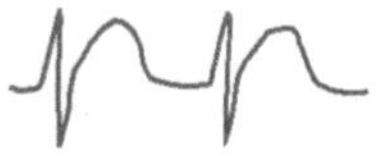 Shortened, almost nonexistent, ST segment causing shortened QT interval
Hypocalcemia	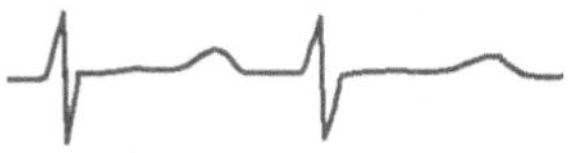 Prolonged ST segment, causing prolonged QT interval

FIGURE 1–23

Miscellaneous effects summary.

chapter one notes TO SUM IT ALL UP . . .

- **Six steps to 12-lead EKG interpretation:**
  - The basics—Rhythm, heart rate, intervals
  - Axis quadrant
  - Bundle branch blocks/hemiblocks
  - Ventricular hypertrophy
  - Miscellaneous effects
  - MI/ischemia
- **Causes of axis deviation:**
  - Normal variant
  - MI
  - Ventricular hypertrophy
  - Arrhythmias
  - Advanced pregnancy or obesity
  - Chronic lung disease, pulmonary embolus
  - Hemiblocks
- **Axis quadrants:**
  - *Normal*—Leads I and aVF both positive, axis 0 to +90 degrees
  - *LAD*—Lead I positive, aVF negative, axis 0 to −90 degrees
  - *RAD*—Lead I negative, aVF positive, axis +90 to ±180 degrees
  - *Indeterminate*—Leads I and aVF both negative, axis −90 to ±180 degrees
- **Right bundle branch block**—RSR' in V_1; QRS ≥0.12 secs. Caused by coronary artery disease, conduction system lesions, right ventricular hypertrophy, congenital heart disease, right ventricular dilatation. Can be normal.

- **Left bundle branch block**—RS or QS in V_1; QRS ≥0.12 secs. Caused by coronary artery disease, hypertension, conduction system lesion, other heart disease. Is *never* normal.
- **Rate–related BBB**—Occurs at a critical rate—when bundle branches can't depolarize fast enough to keep up.
- **Hemiblock**—Block of one of the fascicles of the left bundle branch.
  - *LAHB*—Small Q in Lead I, small R in Lead III, left axis deviation, QRS <0.12 secs
  - *LPHB*—Small R in Lead I, small Q in Lead III, right axis deviation, QRS <0.12 secs
- **Right ventricular hypertrophy**—Tall R in V (≥S wave), right axis deviation; may or may not have inverted T wave
- **Left ventricular hypertrophy**—R wave in V_5 or V_6 + S in V_1 or V_2 ≥ 35
- **Low voltage EKGs caused by:**
  - Obesity
  - Emphysema
  - Myxedema
  - Pericardial effusion
- **Hypertrophy strains the heart and causes ventricular enlargement or dilatation.**
- **Digitalis effect**—Sagging or scooping ST segments
- **Hyperkalemia**—Tall, pointy T waves, then eventually widened QRS complexes
- **Hypokalemia**—Prominent U waves, flattened T waves
- **Hypercalcemia**—Shortened ST segment
- **Hypocalcemia**—Prolonged ST segment

Practice Quiz

1. If the QRS complexes in Leads I and aVF are both negative, in what quadrant is the axis?

   _____

2. True or False. Right bundle branch block almost always implies cardiovascular disease.

3. Sagging ST segments are associated with which miscellaneous effect?

   _____

4. True or False. Tall, pointy T waves are typical of RBBB.

5. Name three causes of axis deviations.

   _____

6. Write the voltage criteria for LVH.

   _____

7. True or False. RVH is always associated with an inverted T wave.

8. Define *hypertrophy*. _____

   _____

9. Hypokalemia has what effect on the T wave?

   _____

10. In a BBB, the QRS interval must be at least _____ seconds.

Putting It All Together—Critical Thinking Exercises

These exercises may consist of diagrams to label, scenarios to analyze, brain-stumping questions to ponder, or other challenging exercises to boost your understanding of the chapter material.

1. If both the right and left bundle branches became blocked simultaneously and no lower pacemaker takes over to control the ventricles, which rhythm would result?

_____

2. Draw the characteristic QRS configuration of a RBBB and a LBBB in V_1.

3. Your patient is a 29-year-old female who has a 6-month-old baby and 8-year-old twins. She had an EKG about 7 months ago and again today. In the first EKG, Lead I was positive and aVF was negative. Today Leads I and aVF are both positive. Explain what happened. _____

_____

_____

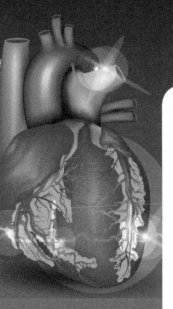

Myocardial Infarction

2

CHAPTER 2 OBJECTIVES

Upon completion of this chapter, the student will be able to

- Describe the difference between ST elevation MI (STEMI) and non-ST elevation MI (NSTEMI).
- State the symptoms of MI.
- Describe the three I's of infarction.
- Describe what EKG changes are associated with ischemia, injury, and infarction.
- Draw the different kinds of ST segment abnormalities and explain what each implies.
- Draw the different T wave abnormalities and explain what each implies.
- Describe how a significant Q wave differs from a normal Q wave.
- Describe normal R wave progression.
- Identify the transition zone in a variety of EKGs.
- Describe the location of the transition zone for clockwise and counterclockwise rotation.

- Describe the EKG changes associated with MI evolution and give the timeline associated with each change.
- Explain how to determine the age of an MI.
- Name the four walls of the left ventricle.
- Name the leads that look at each of the four walls of the left ventricle.
- Describe an easy way to find posterior MIs.
- Name the coronary artery that feeds each of the four walls of the left ventricle.
- Describe how to determine if a right ventricular infarction is present.
- Describe precordial lead placement for a right-sided EKG.
- Describe how pericarditis and early repolarization mimic an MI.
- Describe the EKG complications of MI.
- State the routine treatment for STEMI and NSTEMI.

What It's All About

Mr. Bacon has a nasty case of indigestion. It didn't go away with antacids, and it kept him up all last night even though he propped the head of his bed up with three pillows. Now he's starting to feel nauseated and short-winded. Mr. Bacon calls the doctor's office but can't get an appointment until next month, so he settles down in front of the TV with his bottle of antacid and watches his favorite shows. His daughter stops by after some errands and finds her dad not breathing. She calls 911 and the paramedics arrive and find Mr. Bacon in ventricular fibrillation. They defibrillate him and run an EKG. He's having an MI right now. The paramedics rush Mr. Bacon to the closest hospital that can do percutaneous coronary intervention (PCI) and he's rushed into the cardiac catheterization lab where his blocked coronary artery is ballooned open. He goes to the ICU afterward and learns that his indigestion was not really indigestion. It was chest discomfort often seen—and misinterpreted—with an MI. Mr. Bacon and his daughter are taught the warning signs of an MI. He does well and is released a few days later.

Introduction

Myocardial infarctions (MIs) involve death of myocardial tissue in an area deprived of blood flow by an occlusion (blockage) of a coronary artery. Actual death of tissue is the end of a process that begins with ischemia and injury.

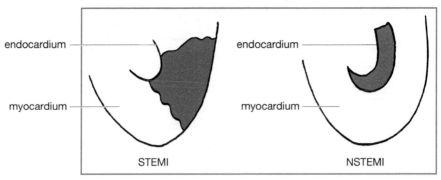

FIGURE 2–1

STEMIs and NSTEMIs.

There are two types of myocardial infarctions: ST elevation MIs (STEMI) and non-ST elevation MIs (NSTEMI).

- STEMIs tend to be transmural (i.e., they usually, though not always, damage the entire thickness of the myocardium in a certain area of the heart). STEMIs result in ST segment elevation, T wave inversion, and significant Q waves, along with the usual symptoms of an MI.
- The NSTEMI tends to be subendocardial or incomplete, damaging only the innermost layer of the myocardium just beneath the endocardium. This kind of MI typically does less damage than a STEMI and does not result in the typical EKG changes associated with STEMIs. NSTEMIs can be difficult to diagnose. They sometimes present with widespread ST segment depression and T wave inversion. At other times, the MI is diagnosed only by patient history, ST segment changes, and elevated lab values that indicate myocardial damage. With NSTEMIs, the patient will have the usual symptoms of an MI and will typically go on to have a STEMI within a few months if treatment for the coronary artery blockage is not provided. See Figure 2–1.

This chapter will focus on recognition of STEMIs, because they are the most common type of MI and require urgent recognition and treatment.

Symptoms of MI

The classic symptom of an MI, whether STEMI or NSTEMI, is chest pain. It is often described as left-sided chest tightness, heaviness, pressure, "an elephant sitting on the chest," or some variation of those. This sensation can even extend into the jaw, the right chest, the neck, the back, or down the arm (usually the left arm). It can even present as a stubborn toothache. See Figure 2–2. Keep in mind that patients with long-time diabetes may not have chest or other discomfort with their MI. They can have a condition called neuropathy, which results in diminished pain sensation. Diabetics are notorious for having "silent MIs," those that show up, perhaps on a routine EKG at the physician's office, without the typical signs and symptoms. Also important to note is that *females in general are more likely to have atypical symptoms when they infarct*. Be suspicious when a female, especially one who is postmenopausal, complains of fatigue, shortness of breath, or other vague symptoms. It could be her version of chest pain—what cardiologists call women's anginal equivalent. (Angina means chest pain.)

Other symptoms of MI are shortness of breath, nausea/vomiting, pallor, diaphoresis, and arrhythmias. Not all patients with MI will have all these symptoms. An unfortunate symptom seen too often with MI is sudden cardiac death from an arrhythmia, usually V-fib. Many individuals with MI never make it to the hospital. For those who do, it is crucial that we offer the best care possible. Let's learn more about MIs.

EARLY SIGNS OF ACUTE CORONARY SYNDROME (HEART ATTACK)

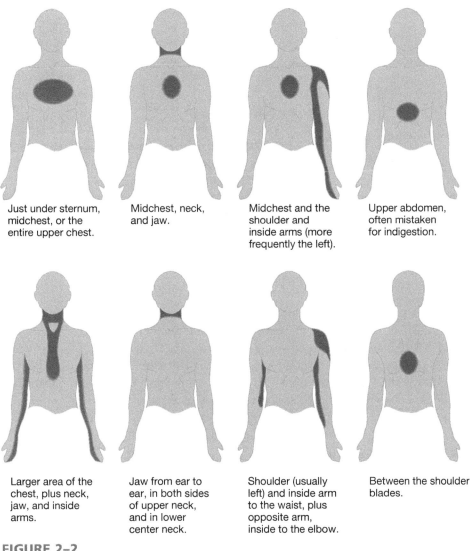

Just under sternum, midchest, or the entire upper chest.

Midchest, neck, and jaw.

Midchest and the shoulder and inside arms (more frequently the left).

Upper abdomen, often mistaken for indigestion.

Larger area of the chest, plus neck, jaw, and inside arms.

Jaw from ear to ear, in both sides of upper neck, and in lower center neck.

Shoulder (usually left) and inside arm to the waist, plus opposite arm, inside to the elbow.

Between the shoulder blades.

FIGURE 2–2

Chest pain locations.

The Three I's of Infarction

The sequence of events that occurs when a coronary artery becomes occluded is known as the *three I's of infarction:*

- Ischemia.   Experiments on dogs have shown that almost immediately after a coronary artery becomes occluded, the *T wave inverts* in the EKG leads overlooking the occluded area. This indicates that myocardial tissue is ischemic, starving for blood and oxygen due to the lack of blood flow. Myocardial tissue becomes pale and whitish in appearance.
- Injury.   As the coronary occlusion continues, the once-ischemic tissue becomes injured by the continued lack of perfusion. The tissue becomes bluish in appearance. The *ST segment rises,* indicating a current of injury and the beginning of an acute STEMI.
- Infarction.   If occlusion persists, the jeopardized myocardial tissue necroses (dies) and turns black. *Significant Q waves develop* (in STEMIs) on the EKG. In time, the dead tissue will become scar tissue.

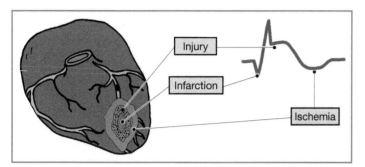

FIGURE 2–3

The three I's of infarction.

Ischemia and injury to myocardial tissue cause repolarization changes, so the ST segments and the T waves will be abnormal. Infarction causes depolarization changes, so the QRS complex will show telltale signs of permanent damage. See Figure 2–3.

In Figure 2–3, an occlusion in a coronary artery is blocking the blood flow to the portion of myocardium fed by that artery. This creates three distinct zones. The innermost zone is the infarcted zone. It is the area that has been deprived of oxygen the longest, as it's the deepest layer and thus farthest away from the blood supply. Immediately surrounding that area is the injured zone, and surrounding that is the ischemic zone.

Ischemia and injury are reversible if circulation is restored. Once the tissue has infarcted, however, the tissue is permanently dead. Myocardial cells do not regenerate.

To determine if an MI is present, we look at the ST segments, the T waves, and the QRS complexes. Let's look at each of those separately.

ST Segment

The normal ST segment should be on the baseline at the same level as the PR segment. (Think of the PR segment as the baseline for ST segment evaluation purposes.) Abnormal ST segments can be elevated or depressed. To see if the ST segment is elevated or depressed, draw a straight line extending from the PR segment out past the QRS. An elevated ST segment is one that is above this line. A depressed ST segment is one that is below this line. *ST segment elevation implies myocardial injury.* ST elevation can be either concave or convex. Convex ST segment elevation (also called a coved ST segment) is most often associated with a STEMI in progress. Concave ST elevation is often associated with pericarditis, an inflammation of the pericardium and the myocardium immediately beneath it, but it can also be seen in STEMIs. *ST depression implies ischemia or reciprocal changes opposite the area of infarct.* See Figure 2–4.

In Figure 2–4, note how the ST segment is right on line with the PR segment in the normal ST example.

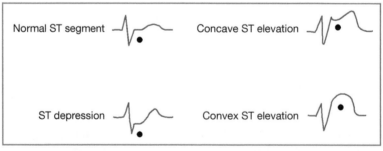

FIGURE 2–4

ST segment abnormalities.

T Wave

The normal T wave should be rounded with an amplitude less than or equal to 5 mm in the frontal leads and should be upright in all leads except aVR and V_1; aVR's T wave should be negative. V_1's T wave can be flat, inverted, or upright. See Figure 2–5.

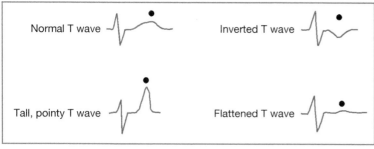

FIGURE 2–5

T wave abnormalities.

All the abnormal T waves in Figure 2–5 can imply myocardial ischemia. The tall, pointy T can also signal hyperkalemia or *hyperacute* changes of an MI in progress. Hyperacute changes are those that accompany an MI in its earliest stages.

QRS Complexes

We look for significant Q waves and poor R wave progression as clues to an MI. Normal Q waves imply septal and right ventricular depolarization. A significant (i.e., pathological) Q wave implies myocardial necrosis. For a Q wave to be significant, it must be *either* 0.04 seconds (one little block) wide *or* at least one-third the size of the R wave. In Figure 2–6, see the difference between a normal Q and a significant Q.

R Wave Progression and Transition

In the precordial leads, you'll recall that the QRS starts out primarily negative in V_1 and goes through a transition around V_3 or V_4, where the QRS is isoelectric. The QRS then ends up primarily positive by V_6. Thus, the R waves progress from very small in V_1 to very large in V_6. If the R waves do not get progressively larger in the precordial leads, as they should, this can imply myocardial infarction. Sometimes poor R wave progression is the only electrocardiographic evidence of an MI.

The transition zone is the lead in which the QRS becomes isoelectric. This transition should occur between V_3 and V_4. A transition in V_1 or V_2 is called counterclockwise; a transition in V_5 or V_6 is clockwise. See Figure 2–7.

In Figure 2–7, look at the R wave progression in the normal transition example. The R waves grow progressively taller across the precordium, and the transition zone is in V_4. See how V_4's QRS complex is mostly isoelectric? Here, V_1 through V_3 are mostly negative, V_5 and V_6 are positive, and V_4 is where the transition from negative to positive occurs.

In the counterclockwise example, the transition zone is between V_1 and V_2. There is no real isoelectric complex. V_1 is negative and V_2 is already positive, so the transition zone would have to be between the two. The R wave progression is abnormal. The R waves progress from very small in V_1 to unusually large in V_2.

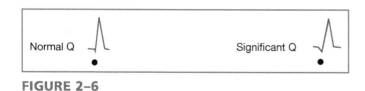

FIGURE 2–6

Normal versus significant Q waves.

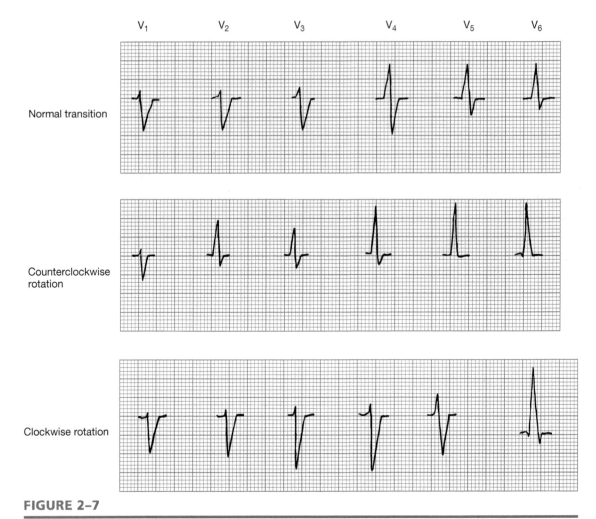

FIGURE 2–7

R wave progression and transition zones in the precordial leads.

In the clockwise example, the transition zone is between V_5 and V_6. R wave progression is abnormal—the R wave is small in V_5 and very tall in V_6.

Evolution of a STEMI

STEMIs occur over a period of time. The EKG changes over the course of a STEMI are its evolution. See Figure 2–8.

Determining the Age of an MI

When an EKG is interpreted, the interpreter does not necessarily know the patient's clinical status and therefore must base determination of the MI's age on the indicative changes present on the EKG. The age of an MI is determined as follows:

- An MI that has ST segment elevation is acute (one to two days old or less).
- An MI with significant Q waves, baseline (or almost back to baseline) ST segments, and inverted T waves is of age indeterminate (several days old, up to a year in some cases). Some authorities call this a **recent MI**.
- The MI with significant Q waves, baseline ST segments, and upright T waves is *old* (weeks to years old).

TIMELINE	AGE OF MI	EKG CHANGE	IMPLICATION
Immediately before the actual MI starts		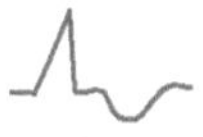 T wave inversion	Cardiac tissue is ischemic, as evidenced by the newly inverted T waves.
Within hours after the MI's start	Acute	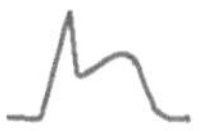 Marked ST elevation + upright T wave	Acute MI has begun, starting with myocardial injury.
Hours later	Acute	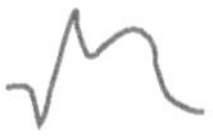 Significant Q + ST elevation + upright T	Some of the injured myocardial tissue has died, while other tissue remains injured.
Hours to a day or two later	Acute	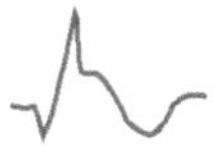 Significant Q + less ST elevation + marked T inversion	Infarction is almost complete. Some injury and ischemia persist at the infarct edges.
Days to weeks later (in some cases this stage may last up to a year)	Age indeterminate	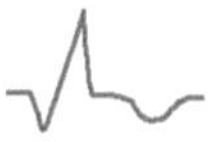 Significant Q + T wave inversion	Infarction is complete. Though there is no more ischemic tissue (it has either recovered or died), the T wave inversion persists.
Weeks, months, years later	Old	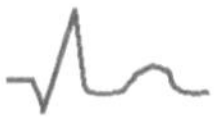 Significant Q only	The significant Q wave persists, signifying permanent tissue death.

FIGURE 2–8

Evolution of a STEMI.

Walls of the Left Ventricle

Although it is possible to have an infarction of the right ventricle, infarctions occur mostly in the left ventricle because it has the greatest oxygen demand and thus is impacted more adversely by poor coronary artery flow. MIs can affect any of the four walls of the left ventricle (see Figure 2–9):

- **Anterior wall.** The front wall—fed by the left anterior descending coronary artery.
- **Inferior wall.** The bottom wall—fed by the right coronary artery.
- **Lateral wall.** The left side wall of the heart—fed by the circumflex coronary artery.
- **Posterior wall.** The back wall—fed by the right coronary artery.

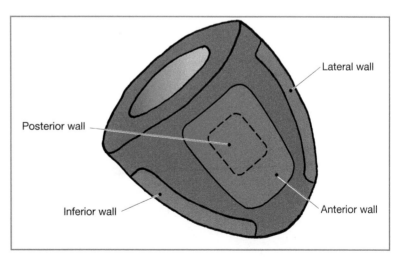

FIGURE 2–9

Walls of the left ventricle.

Each of these left ventricular walls can be "seen" by our EKG electrodes. You'll recall that the positive pole of Leads II, III, and aVF sit on the left leg. They look at

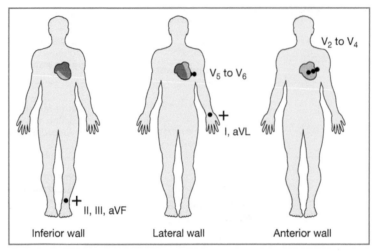

FIGURE 2–10

Leads looking at the anterior, inferior, and lateral walls of the left ventricle.

the heart from the bottom. Which wall of the heart would they see? Good for you if you said the inferior wall.

What about Leads I, aVL, and V_5 and V_6? They sit on the heart's left side, so they look at the lateral wall.

Leads V_2 through V_4 sit right in the front of the heart, looking at the anterior wall. See Figure 2–10.

What about the posterior wall? Unlike the other infarct locations, there are no leads looking directly at the posterior wall because we do not put EKG electrodes on the patient's back for a routine 12-lead EKG. Therefore, the only way to look at the posterior wall is to look *through* the anterior wall. See Figure 2–11.

The ventricles depolarize from endocardium to epicardium (from inside to outside). You'll note on Figure 2–11 that the vectors (arrows) representing depolarization of the anterior and posterior walls are opposite each other. Therefore, *the only way to diagnose a posterior MI is to look for changes opposite those that would be seen with an anterior MI.* We use leads V_1 and V_2 because they sit almost directly opposite the posterior wall. What's the opposite of a Q wave? An R wave. What's opposite ST elevation? ST depression. What's opposite T wave inversion? Upright T wave. Those are what we look for with a posterior infarct.

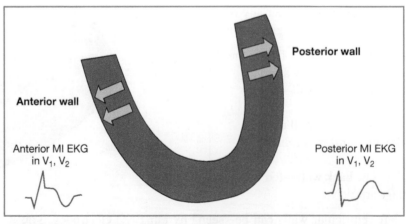

FIGURE 2–11

Posterior wall MI changes.

An easy way to find posterior MIs is to turn the EKG upside down (make the top the bottom) and look at V₁ and V₂ from the back of the EKG. This mimics what the EKG would look like if we had leads directly over the posterior wall. If there is a significant Q wave and T wave inversion in V_1 and V_2 in this upside-down reverse approach, there is a posterior MI. The ST segment may be elevated or at baseline, depending on the age of the MI. Also keep in mind that posterior MIs almost always accompany an inferior MI, so always look for a posterior MI when an inferior MI is present.

Myocardial Infarction Locations

A STEMI is diagnosed on the EKG by indicative changes (i.e., ST elevation, T wave inversion, and significant Q waves) in the leads for that area. Depending on the age of the infarct, not all of those indicative changes will be present.

In the area electrically opposite the infarct area are reciprocal changes (i.e., ST depression). Reciprocal ST depression is seen only when there is ST elevation in the indicative leads.

Let's look at the EKG changes associated with the different infarction locations. It is not necessary to have every single change listed in order to determine the kind of infarction, but most of the criteria should be met. Note the coronary artery involved. See Table 2–1.

The MIs in Table 2–1 involve only one wall of the left ventricle. MIs can extend across into other walls as well. For example, a patient might have an inferior-lateral MI, which would involve the inferior leads as well as the lateral leads. Combination MIs such as this do not always involve every one of the usual leads. For example, an inferior-lateral MI might involve the inferior leads and only a few lateral leads. An anterior-lateral MI might include the anterior leads and only a few lateral leads.

On the next several pages, you'll find helpful ways of determining the kind of MI you're seeing. First there are infarction squares, then MI pictorials, and then an MI algorithm.

TABLE 2–1   Infarction Locations

Location of STEMI	EKG Changes	Coronary Artery
Anterior	Indicative changes in V_2 to V_4 Reciprocal changes in II, III, aVF	Left anterior descending (LAD)
Inferior	Indicative changes in II, III, aVF Reciprocal changes in I, aVL, and V leads	Right coronary artery (RCA)
Lateral	Indicative changes in I, aVL, V_5 to V_6 May see reciprocal changes in II, III, aVF	Circumflex
Posterior	No indicative changes, because no leads look directly at posterior wall Diagnosed by reciprocal changes in V_1 and V_2 (large R wave, upright T wave, and possibly ST depression). Seen as a mirror image of an anterior MI.	RCA or circumflex
Extensive anterior (sometimes called *extensive anterior-lateral*)	Indicative changes in I, aVL, V_1 to V_6 Reciprocal changes in II, III, aVF	LAD or left main
Anteroseptal	Indicative changes in V_1 plus any anterior lead(s) Usually no reciprocal changes	LAD

chapter CHECKUP

We're about halfway through this chapter. To evaluate your understanding of the material thus far, answer the following questions. If you have trouble with them, review the material again before continuing.

Mrs. Uhura has chest pain radiating to her left arm. She is nauseated and short of breath. An EKG shows ST segment elevation in Leads II, III, and aVF.

Lab results are positive for an MI.

1. Is it a STEMI or a NSTEMI?
2. Which wall of the heart is damaged?
3. In which leads would you expect to see reciprocal changes?

Infarction Squares

In Table 2–2, each lead square is labeled with the wall of the heart at which it looks. When you analyze an EKG, note which leads have ST elevation and/or significant Q waves. Then use the infarction squares to determine the type of infarction. For example, if there were ST elevation in Leads II, III, aVF, and V_5 and V_6, you would note that the MI involves inferior and lateral leads. The MI would be inferior-lateral.

Next let's look at some MI pictorials. Ignore the QRS width in these pictorials—the drawings are just to illustrate what these types of MIs look like.

TABLE 2–2   Infarction Squares

I	aVR	V_1	V_4
Lateral	Ignore this lead when looking for MIs	Septal (posterior if mirror image)	Anterior
II	aVL	V_2	V_5
Inferior	Lateral	Anterior (posterior if mirror image)	Lateral
III	aVF	V_3	V_6
Inferior	Inferior	Anterior	Lateral

MI Pictorials

Anterior STEMI

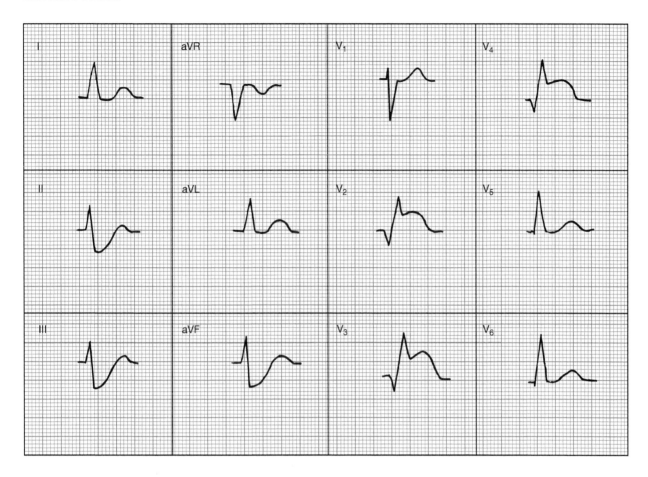

This is an *acute anterior MI*, as evidenced by the ST elevation in V_2 to V_4. Also note the reciprocal ST depression in Leads II, III, and aVF.

If this MI were *age indeterminate,* it would have more normal ST segments, significant Q waves, and T wave inversions in V_2 to V_4.

If this MI were *old* it would have only the significant Q wave remaining. The ST segment would be back at baseline and the T wave would be upright.

Inferior STEMI

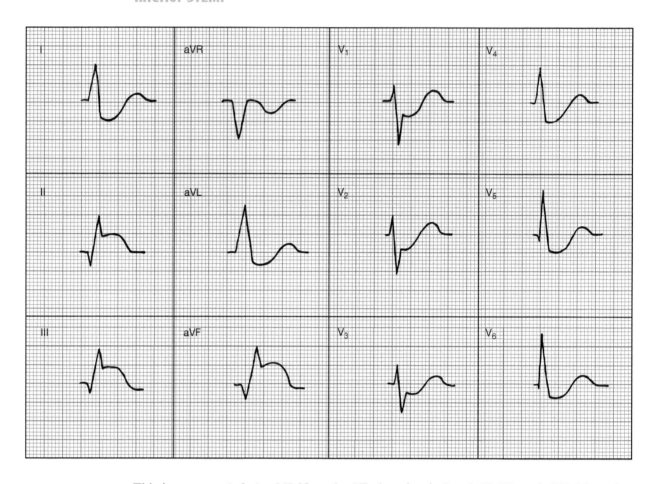

This is an *acute inferior MI*. Note the ST elevation in Leads II, III, and aVF. Note also the reciprocal ST segment depression in Leads I, aVL, and V_1 to V_6.

The *age indeterminate inferior MI* would have more normal ST segments along with significant Q waves and inverted T waves in Leads II, III, and aVF.

The *old inferior MI* would have only significant Q waves in II, III, and aVF. The ST segments would be at baseline and T waves would be upright.

Lateral Wall STEMI

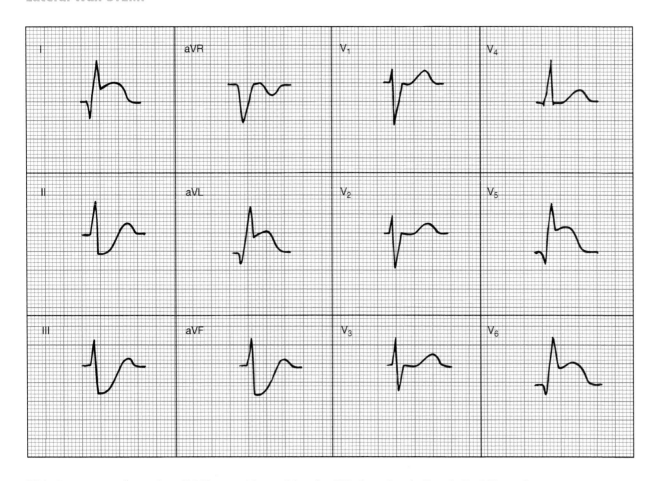

This is an *acute lateral wall MI*, as evidenced by the ST elevation in Leads I, aVL, and V_5 to V_6. Note also the reciprocal ST depression in Leads II, III, and aVF.

If this were an *age indeterminate lateral MI*, there would be more normal ST segments along with significant Q waves and inverted T waves in I, aVL, and V_5 to V_6.

An *old lateral wall MI* would have baseline ST segments, significant Q waves, and upright T waves in I, aVL, and V_5 to V_6.

Posterior MI

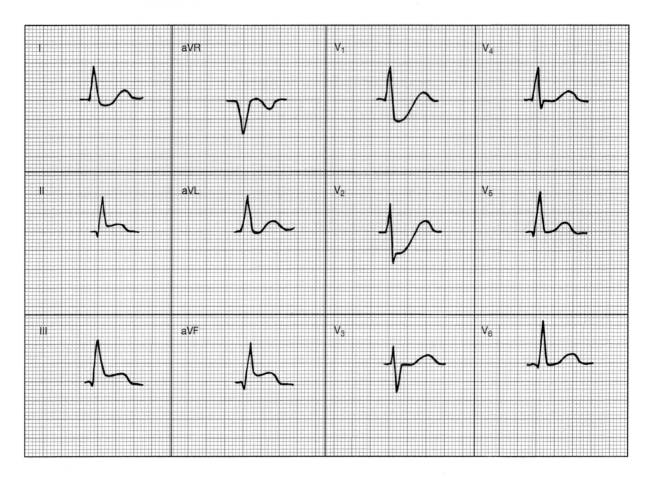

This is an *acute posterior wall MI*. Note the tall R wave in V_1 to V_2 along with ST segment depression and an upright T wave. Remember, a posterior MI is diagnosed by a mirror image of the normal indicative changes of an MI in V_1 to V_2. Note that there is an acute inferior MI as well.

An *age indeterminate posterior MI* would have more normal ST segments, a tall R wave, and an upright T wave.

The *old posterior MI* would have only the tall R wave remaining. The ST segments would be at baseline and the T wave would be inverted.

Extensive Anterior STEMI

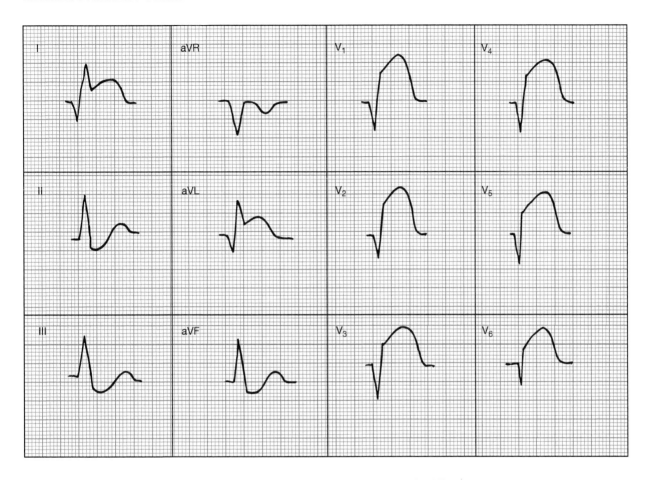

Here we have a huge MI, the *acute extensive anterior MI*. Note the significant Q waves and ST elevation in I, aVL, and V_1 to V_6 along with the reciprocal ST depression in II, III, and aVF.

The *age indeterminate extensive anterior MI* would have more normal ST segments along with significant Q waves and T wave inversion.

The *old extensive anterior MI* would have baseline ST segments, significant Q waves, and upright T waves in I, aVL, and V_1 to V_6.

Anteroseptal STEMI

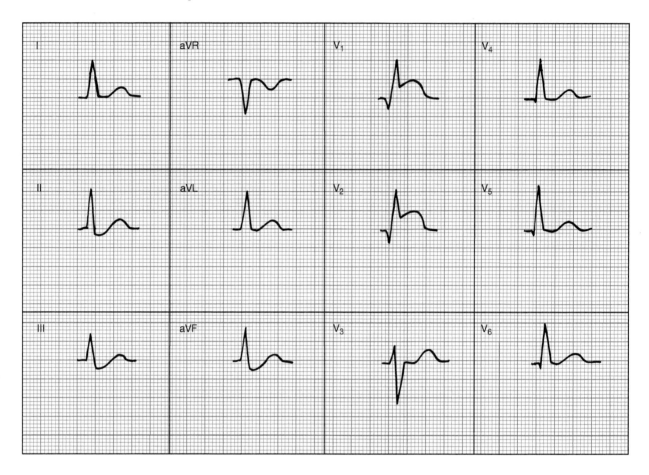

This is an *acute anteroseptal MI*. Note the ST elevation in Leads V₁ to V₂. Recall V₁ is a septal lead and V₂ is an anterior lead. *The combination of V₁ plus any anterior lead results in an anteroseptal MI.*

If this were an *age indeterminate anteroseptal MI,* it would have more normal ST segments, significant Q waves, and inverted T waves in V₁ to V₂.

If this were an *old anteroseptal MI*, it would have only significant Q waves remaining in V₁ to V₂. The ST segments would be at baseline and the T waves would be upright.

NSTEMI

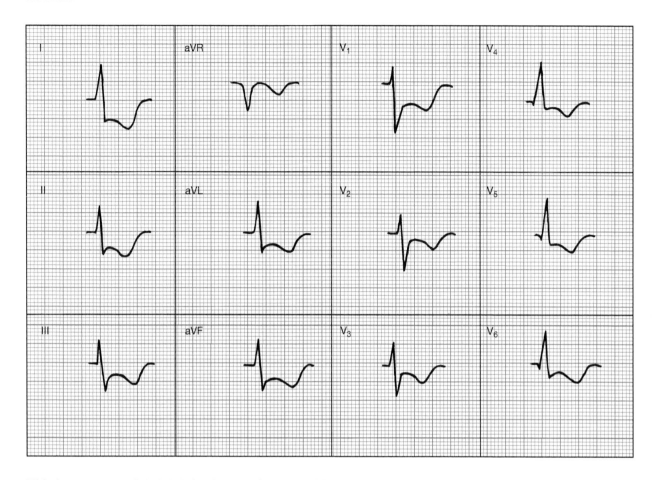

This is an *acute NSTEMI*. It is characterized by widespread ST depression and T wave inversions. NSTEMIs are diagnosed only in the acute phase, as they do not cause significant Q waves, and their T waves are already inverted.

Myocardial Infarction Algorithm

This algorithm (flow chart) is designed to point out the myocardial infarction area. Just answer the questions and follow the arrows.

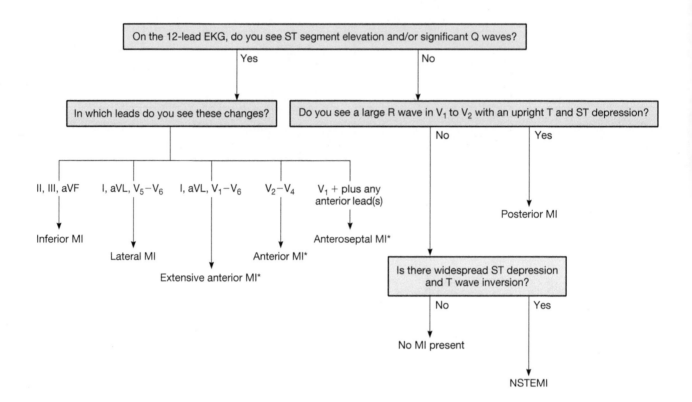

How to Use the MI Algorithm

Refer to the EKG in Figure 2–12. Do you see any ST segment elevation or significant Q waves? Yes, there are significant Q waves, and also there is ST elevation.

In which leads do you see these changes? These are noted in V_1 to V_4. The arrow points to anteroseptal MI.

Right Ventricular Infarction

On occasion, an inferior MI will be accompanied by a right ventricular (RV) infarction. RV infarctions occur when the blockage to the right coronary artery system is so extensive that damage extends into the right ventricle. RV infarctions are not detectable by the routine 12-lead EKG, which looks at the left ventricle. To diagnose an RV infarction, two conditions must be met: First, there must be electrocardiographic evidence of an inferior wall MI on a standard 12-lead EKG. Second, a right-sided EKG must reveal ST elevation in V_3R and/or V_4R. This right-sided EKG is done only if an RV infarction is suspected (i.e., the patient exhibits symptoms, particularly hypotension, beyond what is expected with just an inferior MI).

A right-sided EKG is done with the limb leads in their normal places, but with the precordial leads placed on the right side of the chest instead of the left. See lead placement for a right-sided EKG in Figure 2–13.

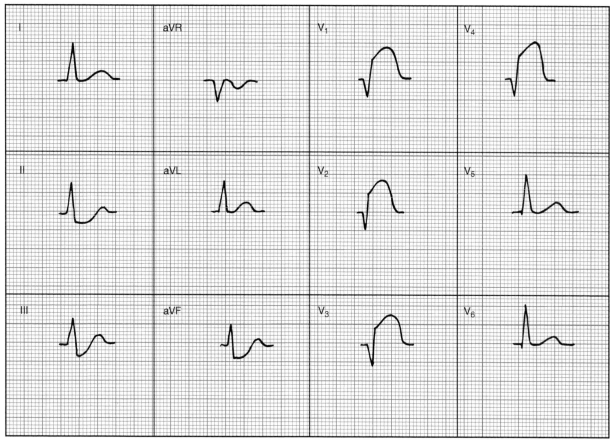

FIGURE 2–12

MI algorithm.

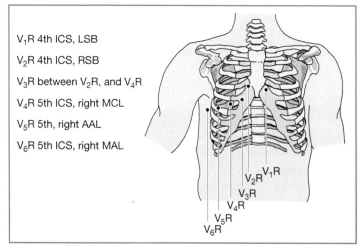

V₁R 4th ICS, LSB

V₂R 4th ICS, RSB

V₃R between V₂R, and V₄R

V₄R 5th ICS, right MCL

V₅R 5th, right AAL

V₆R 5th ICS, right MAL

FIGURE 2–13

Lead placement for a right-sided EKG.

Right Ventricular Infarction (Right-Sided EKG)

See Figure 2–14. On this right-sided EKG, note the ST elevation in Leads V_3R to V_4R. This proves there is an RV infarction. You'll note also that there is ST elevation in Leads II, III, and aVF that indicates an inferior MI. Remember, the right-sided EKG leaves the limb leads in their normal place but moves the precordial leads to the right side of the chest. So the inferior MI will still be obvious on the right-sided EKG.

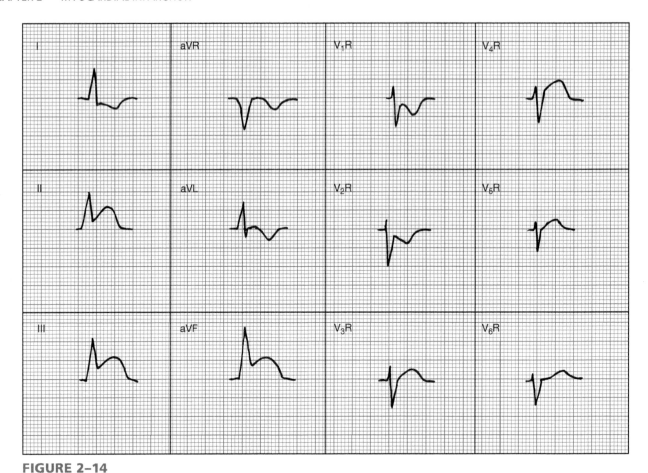

FIGURE 2–14

Right ventricular infarction (right-sided EKG).

Infarct Imposters

Now that you have a feel for the different kinds of MIs, let's look at some conditions that can cause EKG changes that look just like an MI. In most cases, the only difference is in the patient's medical symptoms and history.

Acute Pericarditis

Although ST segment elevation is most often associated with an MI in progress, there are times when it may instead imply an inflammation of the pericardium, called pericarditis. In acute pericarditis, the pericardium and the myocardium just beneath it are inflamed, causing repolarization abnormalities that present as concave ST segment elevation. Because pericarditis does not involve coronary artery blockage, the ST elevation will not be limited to leads overlying areas fed by a certain coronary artery—it will be widespread throughout many leads.

The ST elevation of pericarditis differs from that of an MI in that an MI usually produces *convex* ST elevation, whereas pericarditis produces *concave* elevation. These are often referred to as the *smiley-face* and *frowny-face* ST segments. The smiley face is concave ST elevation. The frowny face is convex. See Figure 2–15.

Like an MI, pericarditis also causes chest pain, and it is crucial to differentiate between the two, as treatment differs greatly. See Figure 2–16.

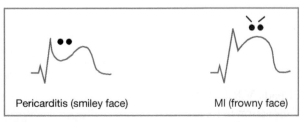

FIGURE 2–15

Smiley-face (concave) and frowny-face (convex) ST elevations.

In Figure 2–16, note the widespread concave ST elevation in Leads I, II, III, aVL, aVF, and V_1 to V_6. This is *not* typical of an MI because it is so widespread. Is it possible this is a huge MI instead of pericarditis? Yes. But based on the concave ST elevation

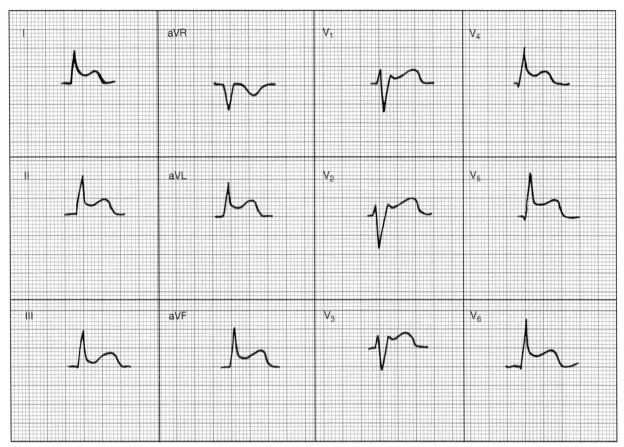

FIGURE 2–16

Pericarditis.

scattered across many leads, it's more likely that it's pericarditis. Only by examining the patient would we know for sure.

Early Repolarization

A normal variant sometimes seen in young people, especially young black males, early repolarization results in ST elevation that may be convex or concave. Repolarization begins so early in this condition that the ST segment appears to start even before the QRS complex has finished, making it appear that the ST segment is mildly elevated. Often there is a "fishhook" at the end of some of the QRS complexes that makes recognition of early repolarization easier. Note the ST elevation and the fishhook (see arrow) in Figure 2–17.

It is not always possible to distinguish early repolarization from an MI based on only a single EKG. A series of EKGs would reveal the typical evolutionary changes if an MI were present, and they would remain unchanged if early repolarization were present. The ST segment elevations of early repolarization are most often evident in Leads V_2 to V_4, although they may be more widespread. Of great help in differentiating early repolarization from an MI is the age and presentation of the patient. A 20-year-old black male with no cardiac complaints who has mild ST elevations probably has early repolarization. A 65-year-old male with chest pain and ST elevation is more likely to have an MI in progress. Only by examining the patient can the definitive diagnosis of early repolarization versus MI be made. See Figure 2–18.

In Figure 2–18, note the mild ST segment elevation in almost all leads and the fishhook in V_3 to V_6 (see arrows). This is typical of early repolarization.

Now it's time for some practice. The EKGs that follow all represent standard left-sided EKGs. The first five EKGs are like the MI pictorials, consisting of only one beat in each lead box. The last five are genuine 12-lead EKGs. Use the infarction squares and/or the MI algorithm if you need help.

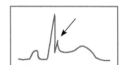

FIGURE 2–17

Fishhook of early repolarization.

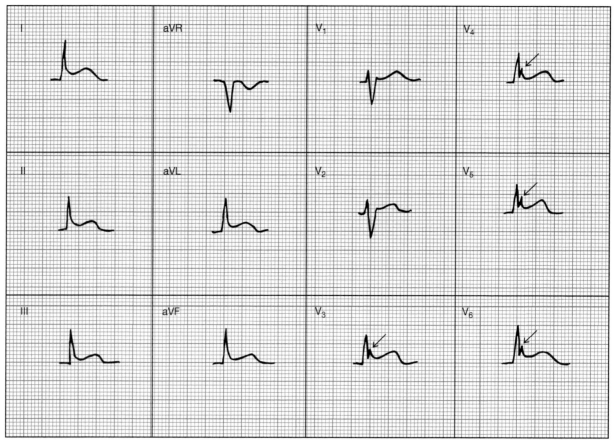

FIGURE 2–18

Early repolarization.

MI Practice

Tell which wall of the heart is affected and how old the MI is (if there is indeed an MI).

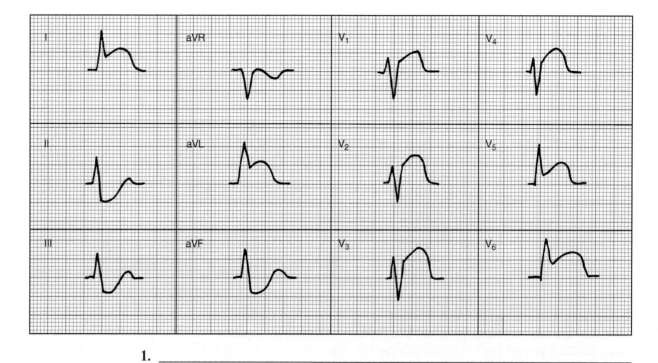

1. _____

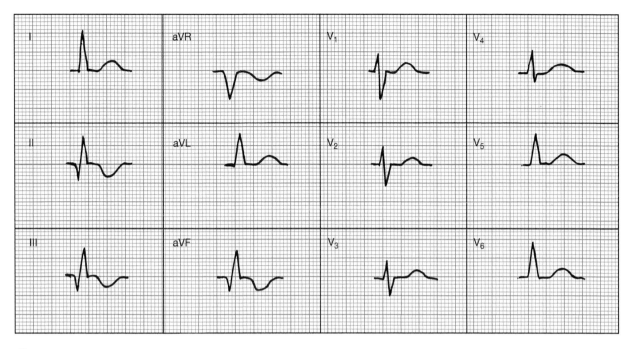

2. _____

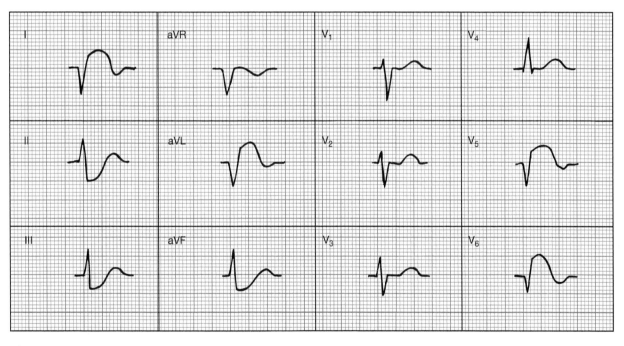

3. _____

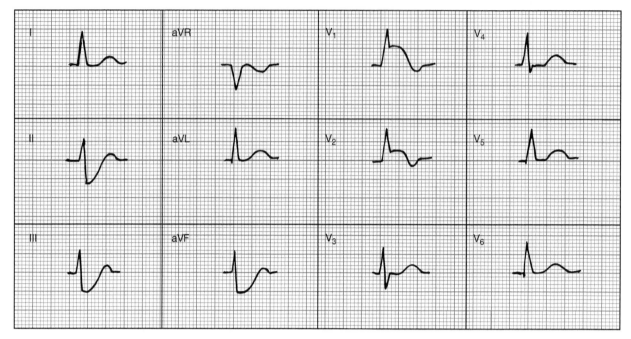

4. _____

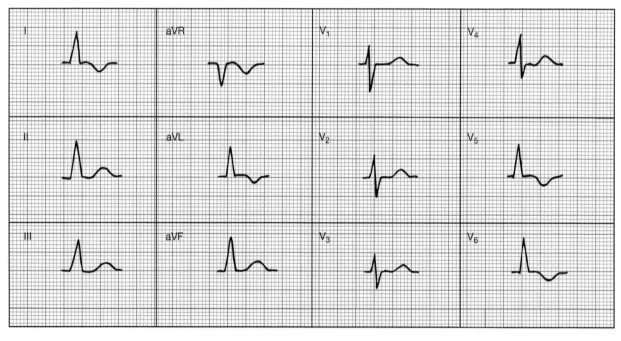

5. _____

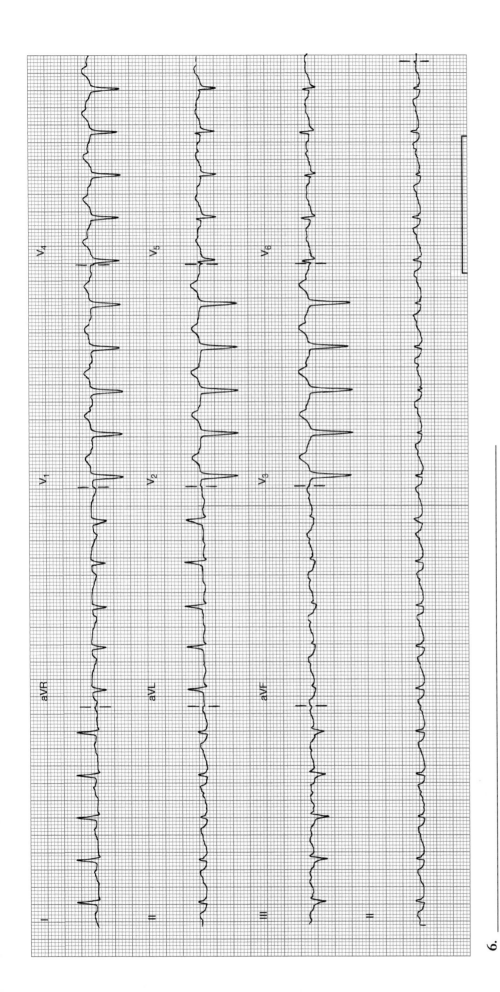

6.

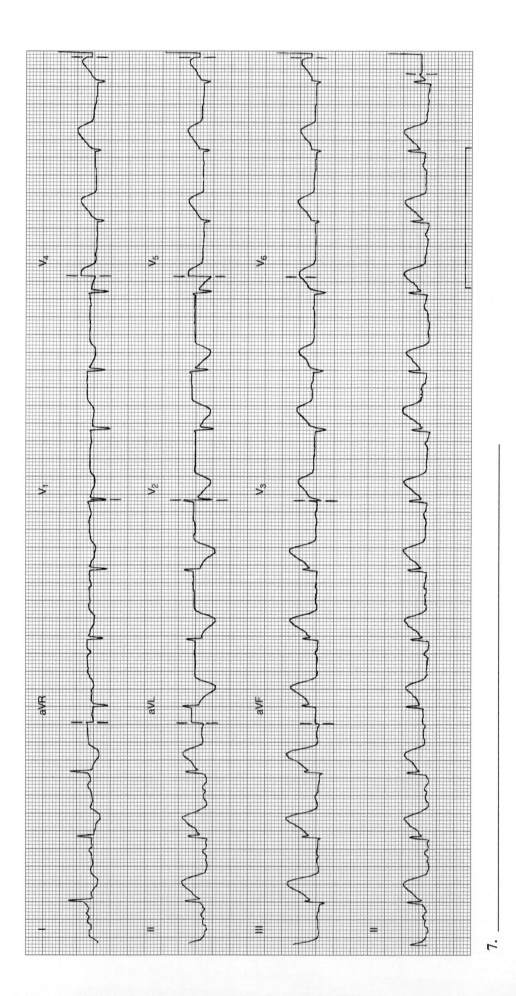

7.

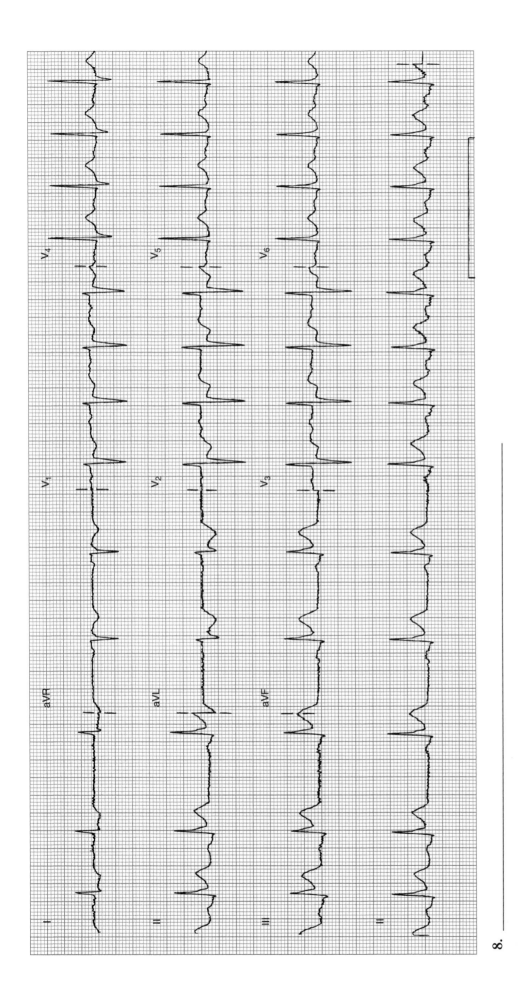

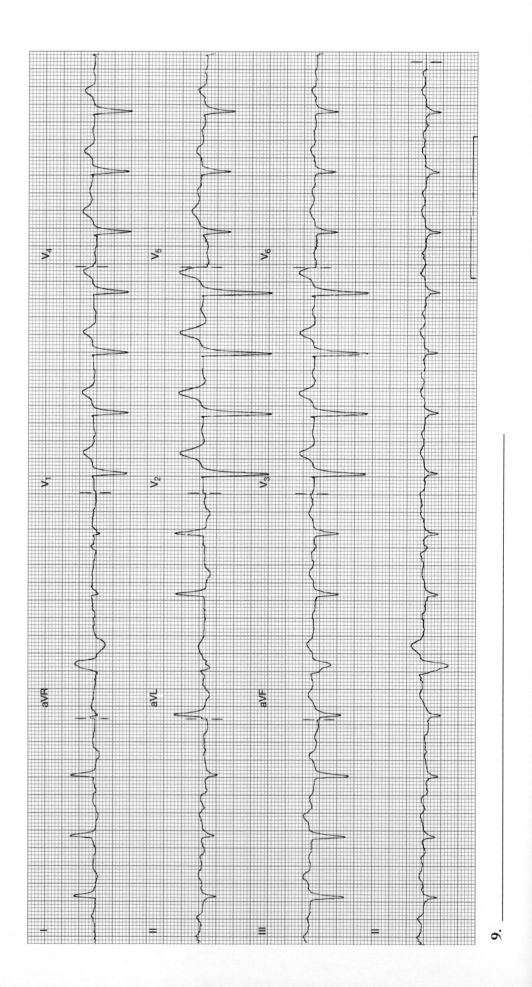

9.

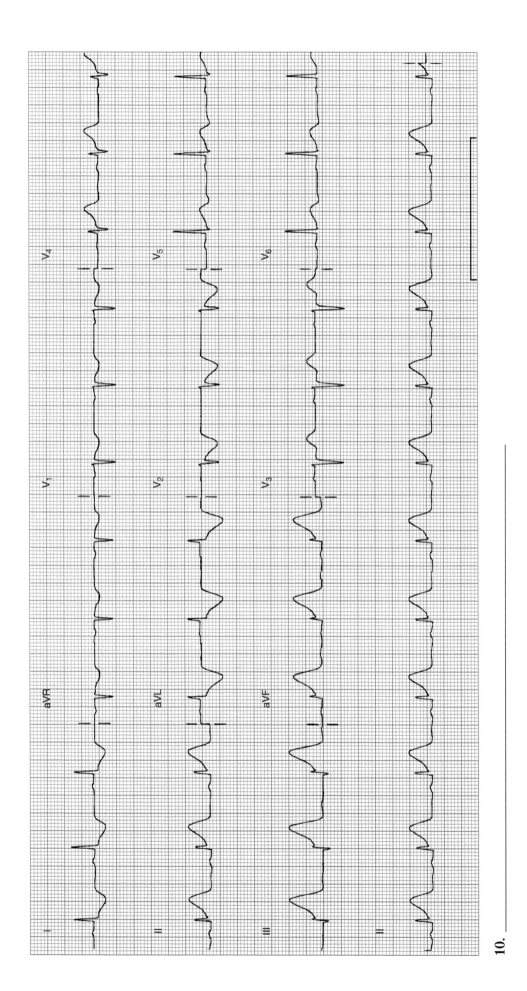

10.

Now that we know how to identify MIs, let's briefly discuss the EKG complications that can occur with the most common MI types—anterior wall MI and inferior wall MI.

Electrocardiographic Complications of MI

Because the myocardium is damaged during an MI, it is not unusual for some degree of heart failure (decreased pumping efficiency) to occur. Because the heart can't pump out as much blood as before, it compensates by pumping more often—this in an attempt to maintain cardiac output. Therefore, sinus tachycardia is common following an MI. Unfortunately this effort by the heart to maintain cardiac output may actually backfire. If the heart rate rises too high, there is not enough time in between beats for the heart to fill up with blood—referred to as decreased diastolic filling time—so the cardiac output drops even more. This can lead to cardiogenic shock, a type of shock caused by catastrophic heart failure.

Arrhythmias are common following MI. Ventricular fibrillation is often seen (and too often fatal) in the first hours after MI and in fact is sometimes the first clue that the person had an MI. The myocardium is very irritable during/after MI and ventricular arrhythmias often result.

Other EKG disturbances occur as well. See Table 2–3 for EKG complications of the most common types of MIs—the anterior and inferior wall MIs.

So now that we can identify MIs and their electrocardiographic complications, how do we treat the MI?

Treatment of MI

Patients suspected of having an MI should have a 12-lead EKG and blood drawn to determine if an MI is in progress. Certain enzymes (Troponin and CPK in particular) are released into the bloodstream by damaged myocardial cells during an MI and can be noted on lab values. Patients will be started on oxygen by nasal cannula to decrease the heart's workload. They'll be given *nitroglycerin* and perhaps *morphine* for chest pain. The nitroglycerin dilates (opens up) the narrowed coronary artery, allowing more blood flow to the stricken myocardium. This can relieve the pain. If that is ineffective, morphine, a narcotic that has cardiac benefits (it modestly decreases return of venous blood to the heart, helping treat/prevent heart failure) can be used to relieve MI pain. Pain is dangerous for the MI patient, because it increases heart rate and stresses the heart even more. Relieving pain is extremely important. MI patients will be given an *aspirin* to chew (yes, chew) to help decrease platelet aggregation (clumping of platelets). Platelet aggregation forms clots. Preventing this aggregation helps prevent any blood clot that is already in the coronary artery from growing larger. *These meds are given only if there are*

TABLE 2–3 EKG Complications of MI

MI WALL	Electrocardiographic Complications
Anterior	Mobitz II second degree AV block, third-degree AV block with wide QRS, bundle branch blocks, sinus tachycardia, ventricular arrhythmias, V-fib in the first hours after infarct, AIVR, right bundle branch block, left posterior hemiblock
Inferior	Bradycardias, first-degree AV block, Wenckebach, ventricular arrhythmias, V-fib in the first hours after infarct, accelerated junctional rhythm, junctional bradycardia, AIVR, third-degree AV block with narrow QRS
Anteroseptal	Same as anterior, with increased chance of V-fib occurring greater than 48 hours after MI

no contraindications. For example, a patient with bleeding ulcers in his or her stomach may not be given the aspirin, because it would increase the chance of bleeding. The above combination of meds is referred to as *MONA: morphine-oxygen-nitro-aspirin.*

Treatment of STEMIs and NSTEMIs differs after initial treatment and diagnostic workup. NSTEMIs are treated less aggressively early on, because these MIs do still allow some coronary artery flow distal to (beyond) the narrowed area. NSTEMI patients may receive antiplatelet or anticoagulant medications to thin the blood and prevent recurrences of the MI. They may be started on beta blockers to decrease the heart's workload, and they will likely eventually have an angiogram done to determine the location of the coronary artery blockage. Further treatment can then be determined based on the angiogram results.

Treatment of STEMIs is more emergent than treatment of NSTEMIs because the coronary artery blockage is complete, and myocardial necrosis is a certainty without treatment. The American Heart Association and American College of Cardiology recommend that STEMI patients arriving in the emergency department be taken immediately to the cardiac catheterization lab for reperfusion via PCI (percutaneous coronary intervention), a balloon procedure to open the blocked coronary artery. A wire mesh called a stent may then be placed at the site of the former blockage to serve as a sort of scaffold to keep the artery open. The goal of PCI is a door-to-balloon time of 90 minutes, meaning the STEMI patient should be having the PCI procedure within 90 minutes of arrival at the hospital. At some smaller hospitals without cardiac catheterization labs, PCI is not possible, so STEMI patients at these facilities can either be transported to a nearby facility that can do the PCI within the 90 minutes or they can be treated with thrombolytic medications (medications that dissolve blood clots) within 30 minutes of arrival at the smaller hospital. Thrombolytics dissolve the blood clot causing the MI, but they can be given only to a closely screened population of patients because of the increased risk of bleeding, which can cause strokes or other complications.

Patients with an uncomplicated course following their MI may be home from the hospital in less than a week.

chapter two notes TO SUM IT ALL UP . . .

- **MI**—Death of myocardial tissue—caused by occlusion of a coronary artery.
- **Two types of MI:**
  - *STEMI*—ST elevation MI
  - *NSTEMI*—Non-ST elevation MI
- **Symptoms of MI** (patient may have any or all of these):
  - Chest pain, pressure, or discomfort that can radiate to the arms, jaw, neck, back
  - Pallor
  - Nausea
  - Feeling of impending doom
  - Shortness of breath
  - Lightheadedness or dizziness
- **Females and diabetics are notorious for having atypical symptoms (or no symptoms at all) of their MI.**
- **Three I's of infarction:**
  - *Ischemia*—Decreased blood flow to heart muscle—tissue pale whitish—inverted T wave on EKG.
  - *Injury*—Tissue injured by continued lack of blood flow—tissue bluish—ST segment elevation.

- *Infarction*—Tissue dies and turns black—significant Q waves.
- **ST segment**—Convex (coved) implies STEMI. Concave seen with pericarditis.
- **Hyperacute T waves**—Unusually tall T waves seen in earliest stages of MI.
- **Significant Q wave**—Must be at least 0.04 seconds wide or one-third the size of the R wave.
- **R wave progression**—R waves start out small in V_1 and get larger as they move toward V_6. Transition zone V_3 to V_4.
- **Age of STEMI:**
  - *Acute* = ST elevation
  - *Age indeterminate* = Significant Q wave, ST back (or almost back) to baseline, T wave inverted
  - *Old* = Significant Q wave, ST at baseline, T wave upright
- **Walls of left ventricle:**
  - *Anterior*—Fed by left anterior descending coronary artery
  - *Inferior*—Fed by right coronary artery
  - *Lateral*—Fed by circumflex
  - *Posterior*—Fed by right coronary artery

■ **STEMI criteria:**
- *Anterior* MI—ST elevation V_2 to V_4
- *Inferior*—ST elevation II, III, aVF
- *Lateral*—ST elevation I, aVL, V_5 to V_6
- *Posterior*—ST depression and large R wave in V_1 to V_2
- *Extensive anterior*—ST elevation I, aVL, all V leads
- *Anteroseptal*—ST elevation V_1 plus any other lead from V_2 to V_4

■ **Right ventricular infarction**—Accompanies inferior wall MI—diagnosed by seeing ST elevation in V_3 to V_4R on right-sided EKG.

■ **Pericarditis**—Inflammation of pericardial sac—also inflames myocardium—causes concave ST elevation (smiley face). ST elevation widespread.

■ **Early repolarization**—Common in young people, especially young black males—causes mild ST elevation—sometimes see "fishhook" at end of QRS complexes in the V leads.

■ **EKG Complications of MI:**
- *Anterior MI*—Mobitz II second-degree AV block, third-degree AV block with wide QRS, V-fib in early hours, RBBB, LPHB, AIVR, sinus tachycardia, ventricular arrhythmias
- *Inferior MI*—Bradycardias, first-degree AV block, Wenckebach, third-degree AV block with narrow QRS, accelerated junctional rhythm, junctional bradycardia, AIVR, ventricular arrhythmias, V-fib in early hours
- *Anteroseptal*—Same as anterior but with increased chance of V-fib occurring late (greater than 48 hours after infarct)

■ **MI treatment:**
- *All suspected MIs*—MONA (morphine-oxygen-nitroglycerin-aspirin)
- *STEMI*—PCI or thrombolytics
- *NSTEMI*—Medications such as beta blockers, anticoagulants or anti-platelet agents, eventual angiogram

Practice Quiz

1. List the three I's of infarction. _____
_____
_____

2. State the differences between a STEMI and a NSTEMI. _____
_____

3. Which coronary artery's occlusion results in an anterior wall MI? _____
_____

4. Name the three normal indicative changes of an MI.
_____
_____
_____

5. Reciprocal changes are seen in which area of the heart? _____
_____

6. If there is marked ST elevation in Leads II, III, and aVF, how old is the MI and in which wall of the heart?
_____
_____

7. If there is a significant Q wave in V_1 to V_3 with baseline ST segments and upright T waves, how old is the MI and in which wall of the heart? _____
_____
_____

8. If the transition zone of the precordial leads is in V_1 to V_2, which kind of rotation is the heart said to have? _____
_____

9. The kind of MI that can be diagnosed by inverting the EKG and looking at Leads V_1 and V_2 from behind is the _____
_____

10. Which coronary artery supplies the lateral wall of the left ventricle? _____
_____

Putting It All Together—Critical Thinking Exercises

These exercises may consist of diagrams to label, scenarios to analyze, brain-stumping questions to ponder, or other challenging exercises to boost your understanding of the chapter material.

1. Draw and label the evolution of EKG changes seen from immediately before the actual STEMI starts to a STEMI that is weeks, months, or years old.

2. If Mr. Milner, a 69-year-old man with a history of chest pain, arrives in your ER with newly inverted T waves in Leads II, III, and aVF, what do you suspect is happening _____

   _____

3. If an hour later Mr. Milner is doubled over with crushing chest pain and his EKG now shows marked ST elevation in II, III, aVF and V_5 to V_6, what is happening? _____

   _____

   _____

The following is a scenario that will provide you with information about a fictional patient and ask you to analyze the situation, answer questions, and decide on appropriate actions.

Mr. Jones is a 79-year-old black male who arrives in the ER stating he'd had chest pain for about a half hour prior to arrival, but right now the pain is gone. See his EKG in Figure 2–19.

4. What do you see in Leads II, III, and aVF that would be consistent with myocardial ischemia? _____

   _____

The ER physician orders lab work and the nurse keeps a close eye on Mr. Jones. Thirty minutes later, Mr. Jones calls his nurse, complaining of crushing chest pain and shortness of breath. His blood pressure has dropped and his skin is ashen, cool, and clammy. The nurse calls for the physician and repeats an EKG. See Figure 2–20.

5. What is happening? _____

   _____

The physician orders medication for the pain and sends Mr. Jones to the cath lab for PCI. Within the hour, Mr. Jones feels much better and his EKG is much improved. He is sent to the coronary care unit for a few days and does well.

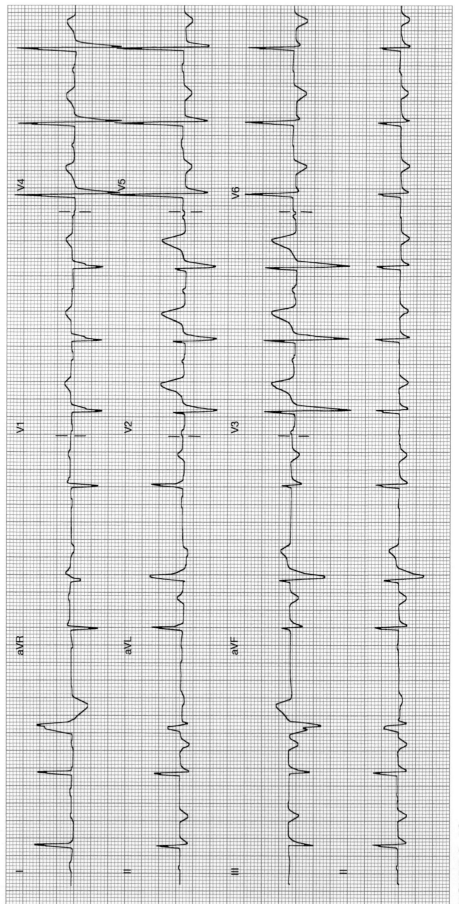

FIGURE 2-19

Mr. Jones's first EKG.

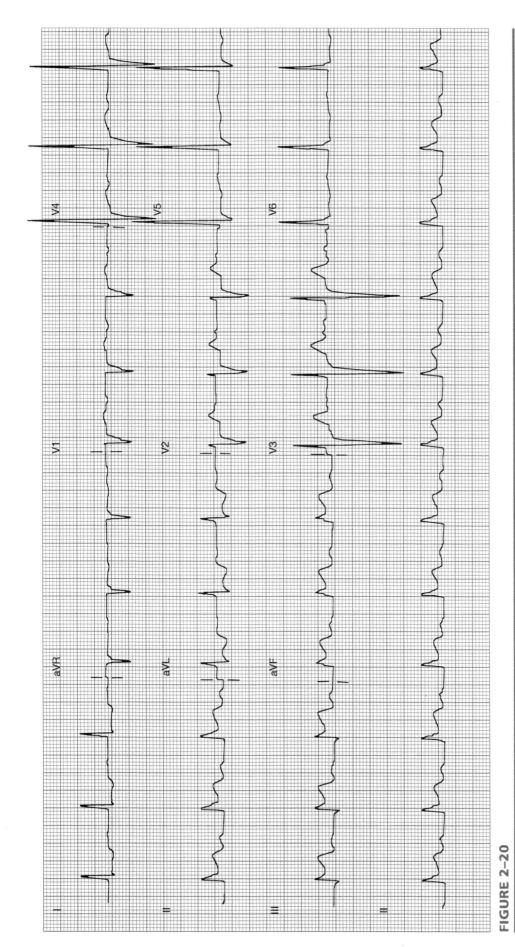

FIGURE 2-20

Mr. Jones's second EKG.

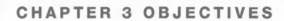

CHAPTER 3 OBJECTIVES

Upon completion of this chapter, the student will be able to

- Utilize the six steps in analyzing EKGs.

- Using this method, correctly interpret a variety of 12-lead EKGs.

What It's All About

Mamie was a new paramedic in orientation with Jake, a paramedic with 12 years of experience. Their first call was for a 65-year-old female complaining of chest pain. The 12-lead EKG looked suspicious to Mamie. "She looks like she's infarcting," whispered Mamie to her co-worker, "Look at that ST segment elevation." Jake agreed. The duo started the patient on oxygen, assessed her vital signs, gave sublingual nitroglycerin, and called in their report to the closest hospital that had a cardiac cath lab capable of performing PCI. They transmitted the EKG to the receiving hospital. When the paramedics arrived at the emergency room with the patient, the cath lab team was standing by to take the patient for PCI. As a result of their recognition that an MI was in progress, the patient received immediate definitive treatment and her MI was minimized in size.

Introduction

This chapter pulls together everything you've learned so far about rhythm and 12-lead EKG interpretation. First, you will find a comprehensive summary of what to look for on every EKG, then a checklist. Refer to these when evaluating the 12-lead EKGs that follow.

There are 20 EKGs to interpret in this chapter. Take your time and be methodical. Don't hesitate to go back and review portions of this text if you find that you're a little weak in certain areas. Practice does indeed make perfect.

12-Lead EKG Interpretation in a Nutshell

You've learned all the criteria for 12-lead EKG interpretation. Let's put it all in condensed form. Look for the following on every 12-lead EKG:

The Basics	Rhythm, Rate, Intervals (PR, QRS, QT)
Axis quadrant	Normal, LAD, RAD, or indeterminate?
BBB/Hemiblock	RBBB = RSR' in V_1, QRS ≥ 0.12 seconds
	LBBB = QS or RS in V_1, QRS ≥ 0.12 seconds
	LAHB = small Q in I, small R in III, left axis deviation
	LPHB = small R in I, small Q in III, right axis deviation
Hypertrophy	RVH = R ≥ S in V_1, right axis deviation; inverted T may or may not be present
	LVH = S in V_1 or V_2 + R in V_5 or V_6 ≥ 35
Miscellaneous	Digitalis effect = Sagging ST segments, prolonged PR interval
	Hyperkalemia = Tall, pointy, narrow T waves
	Severe hyperkalemia = Wide QRS complex
	Hypokalemia = Prominent U waves, flattened T waves
	Hypercalcemia = Shortened ST segment causing short QT interval
	Hypocalcemia = Prolonged ST segment causing prolonged QT interval
Infarction	Anterior MI = ST elevation and/or significant Q in V_2 to V_4
	Inferior MI = ST elevation and/or significant Q in II, III, aVF
	Lateral MI = ST elevation and/or significant Q in I, aVL, V_5 to V_6
	Anteroseptal MI = ST elevation and/or significant Q in V_1 plus any anterior lead
	Extensive anterior (extensive anterior-lateral) = ST elevation and/or significant Q in I, aVL, V_1 to V_6
	Posterior MI = Large R + upright T in V_1 to V_2; may also have ST depression
	Non-ST elevation MI = Widespread ST depression and T wave inversion in many leads
	Ischemia = Inverted T waves in any lead, as long as not BBB-related

12-Lead EKG Interpretation Checklist

The Basics

- Rhythm _____
- Rate _____
- Intervals: PR _____ QRS _____ QT _____

Axis

Circle one:

- Normal
- Abnormal (what quadrant?) _____

Bundle Branch Blocks/Hemiblocks

Circle if present:

- RBBB
- LAHB

- LBBB
- LPHB

Hypertrophy

Circle if present:

- RVH
- LVH

Infarction/Ischemia

Circle if present:

- Infarction
- Ischemia

Which walls of the heart? _____

Miscellaneous Effects

Circle if present:

- Digitalis effect
- Severe hyperkalemia
- Hypercalcemia

- Hyperkalemia
- Hypokalemia
- Hypocalcemia

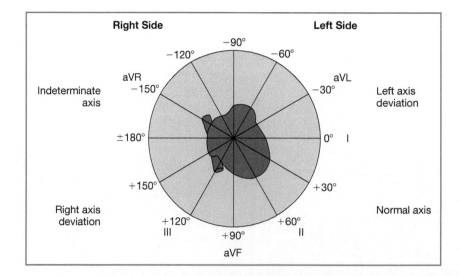

Practice EKGs

1. Rhythm and rate _____ PR _____ QRS _____ QT _____

   Axis _____ BBB/HB _____

   Hypertrophy _____

   Miscellaneous effects _____

   Infarction _____

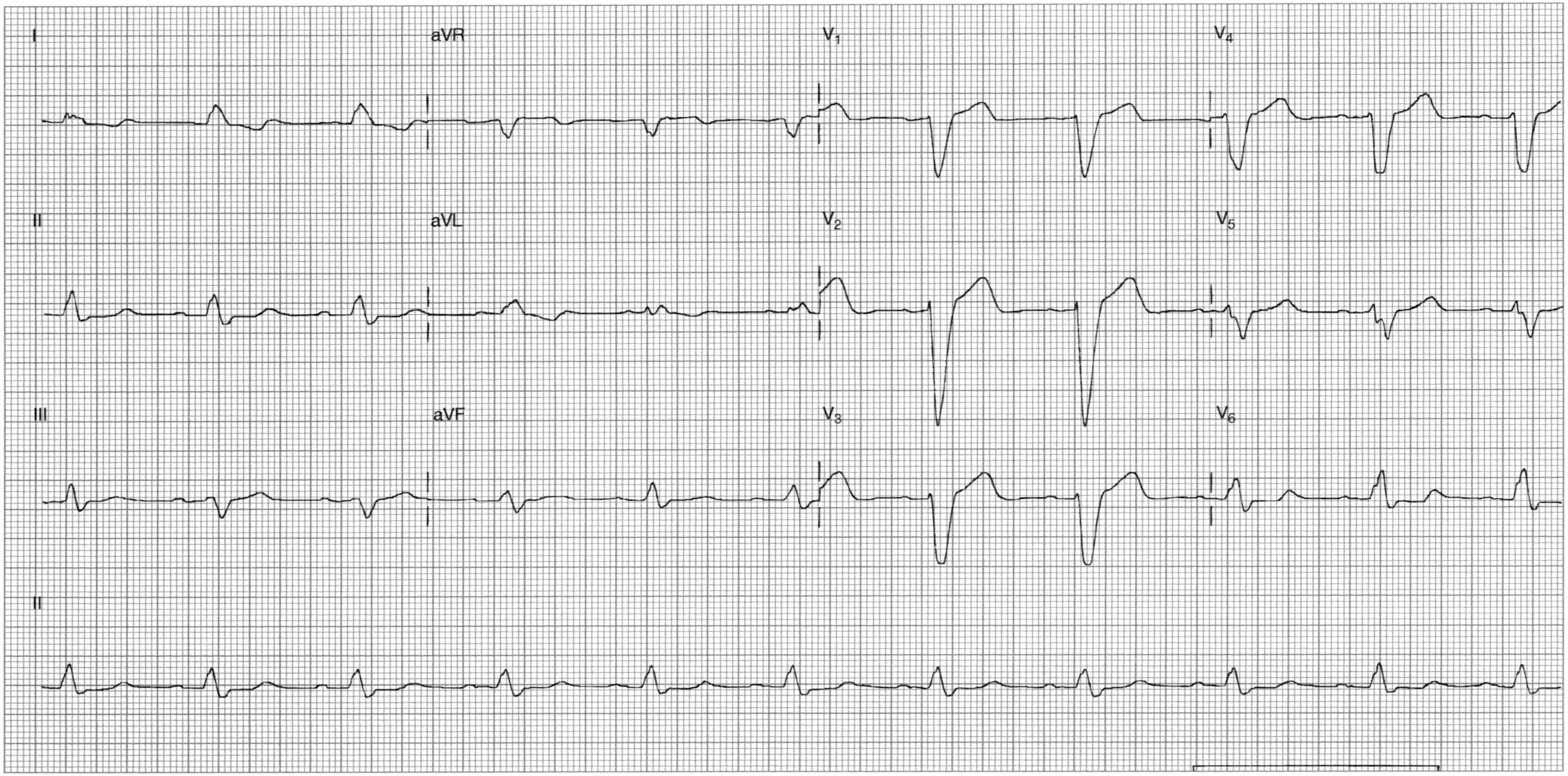

2. Rhythm and rate _____ PR _____ QRS _____ QT _____

Axis _____ BBB/HB _____

Hypertrophy _____

Miscellaneous effects _____

Infarction _____

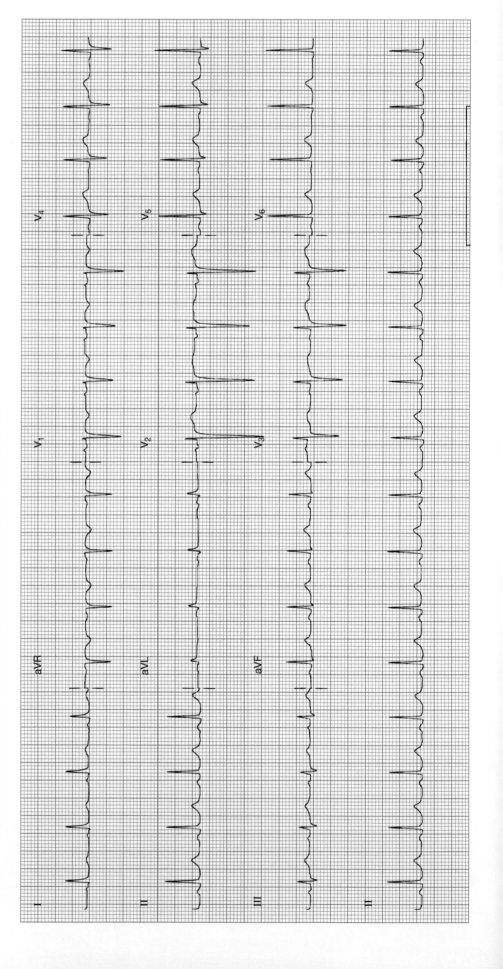

3. Rhythm and rate _____ PR _____ QRS _____ QT _____

Axis _____ BBB/HB _____

Hypertrophy _____

Miscellaneous effects _____

Infarction _____

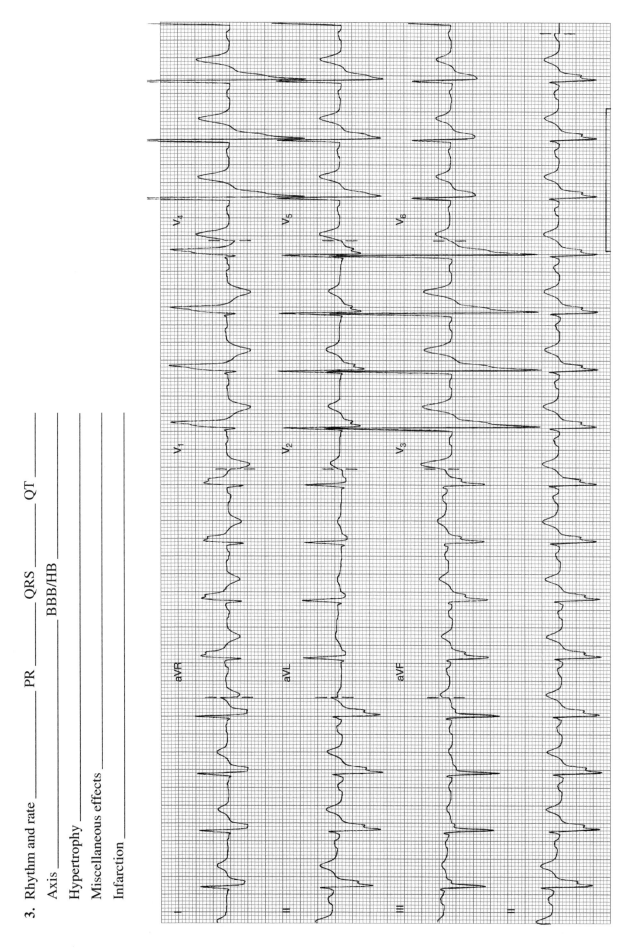

4. Rhythm and rate _____ PR _____ QRS _____ QT _____

Axis _____ BBB/HB _____

Hypertrophy _____

Miscellaneous effects _____

Infarction _____

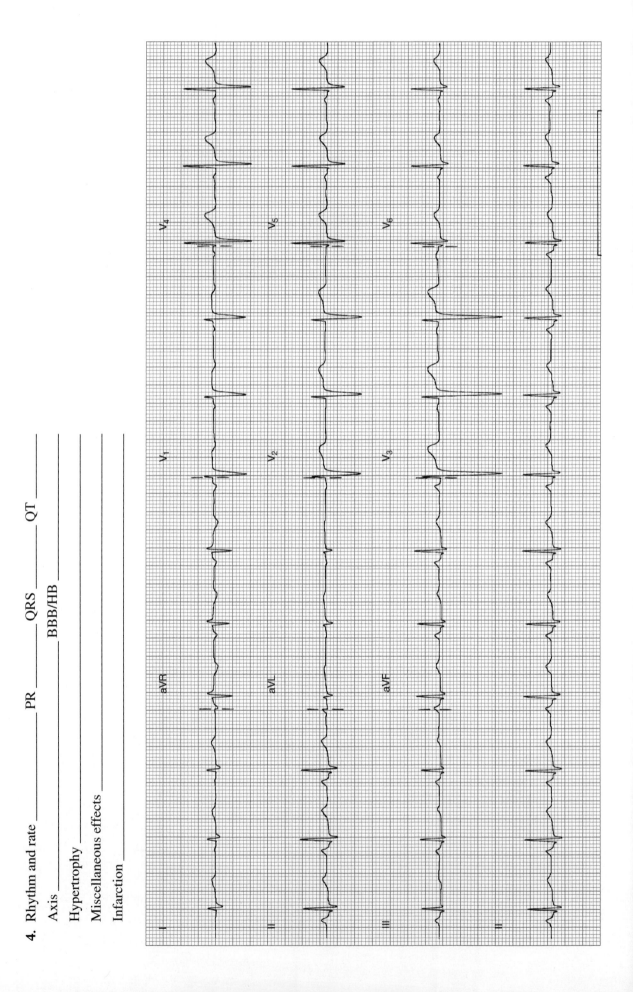

5. Rhythm and rate _____ PR _____ QRS _____ QT _____

Axis _____ BBB/HB _____

Hypertrophy _____

Miscellaneous effects _____

Infarction _____

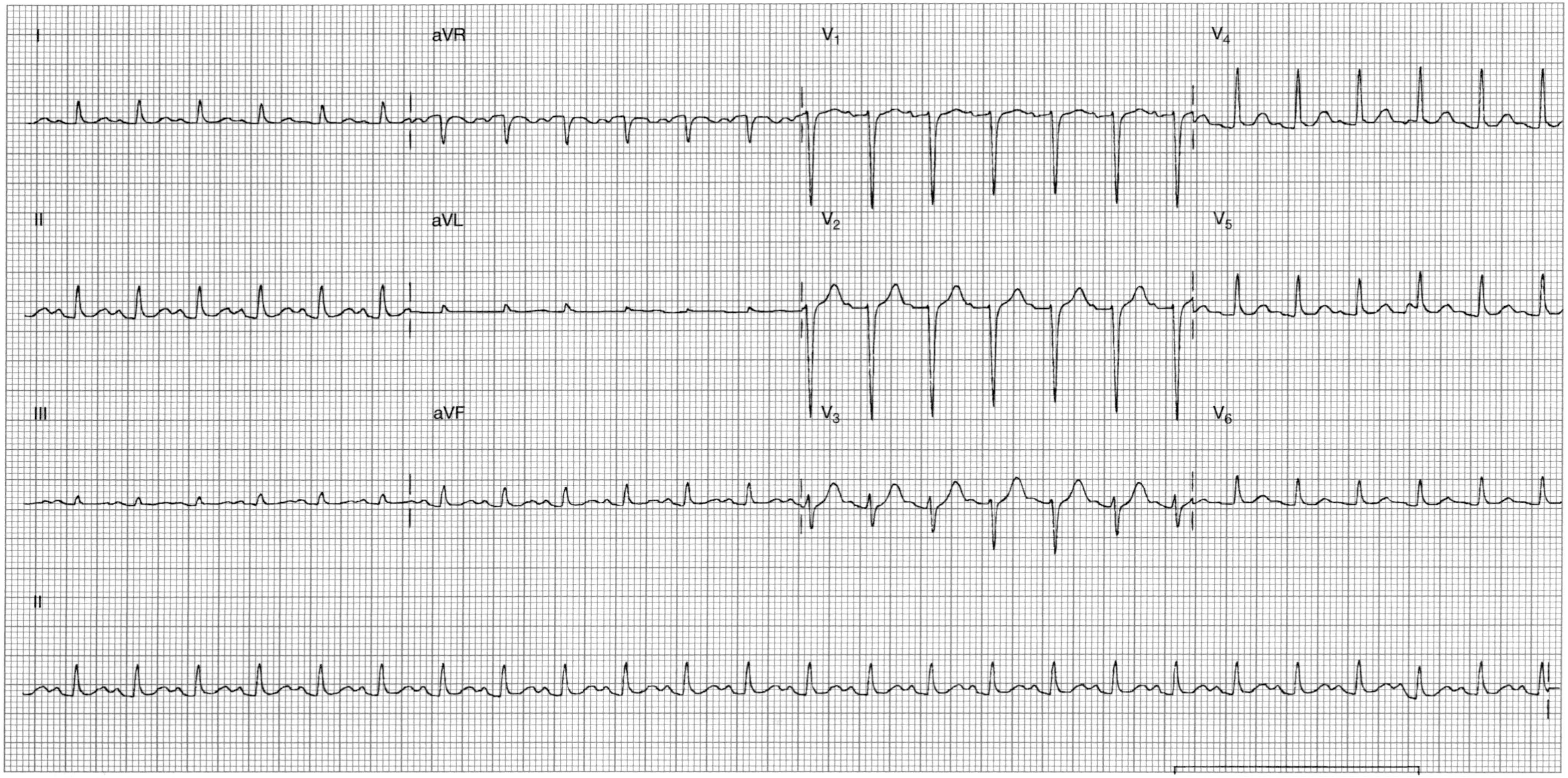

6. Rhythm and rate _____

Axis _____

PR _____ QRS _____ QT _____

_____ BBB/HB _____

Hypertrophy _____

Miscellaneous effects _____

Infarction _____

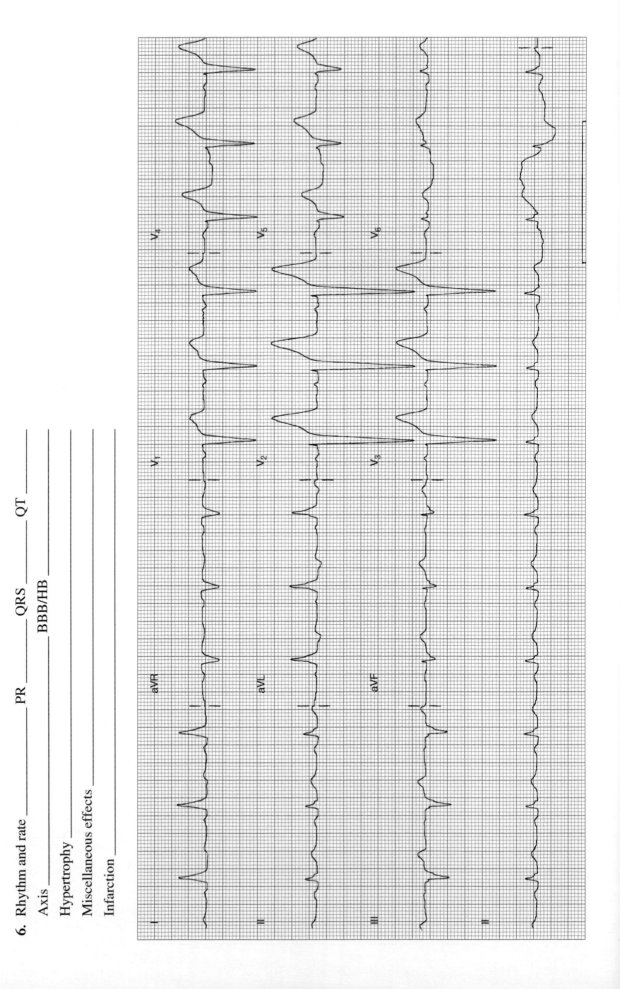

7. Rhythm and rate _____ PR _____ QRS _____ QT _____

Axis _____ BBB/HB _____

Hypertrophy _____

Miscellaneous effects _____

Infarction _____

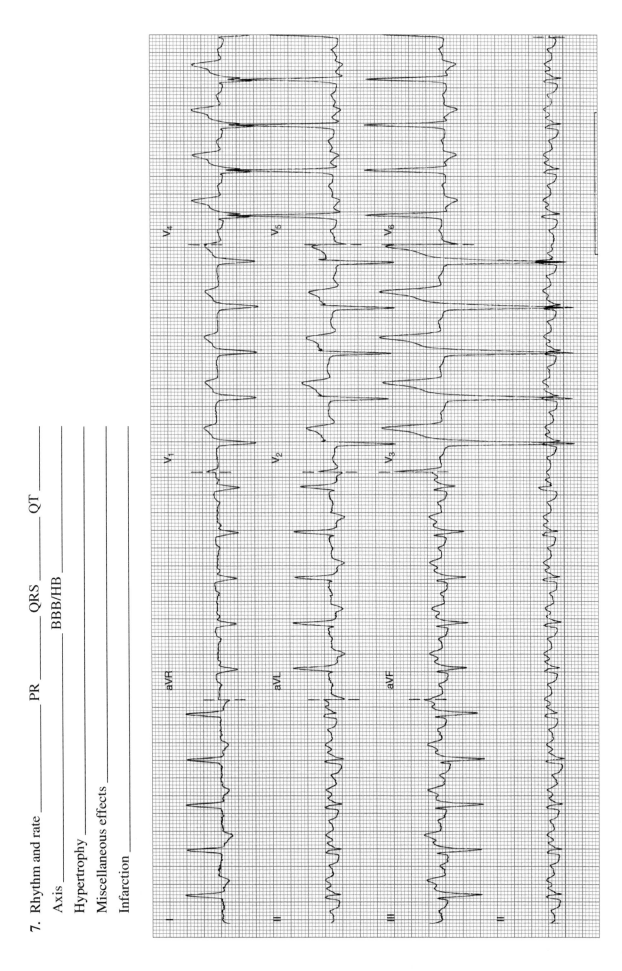

8. Rhythm and rate _____ PR _____ QRS _____ QT _____

Axis _____ BBB/HB _____

Hypertrophy _____

Miscellaneous effects _____

Infarction _____

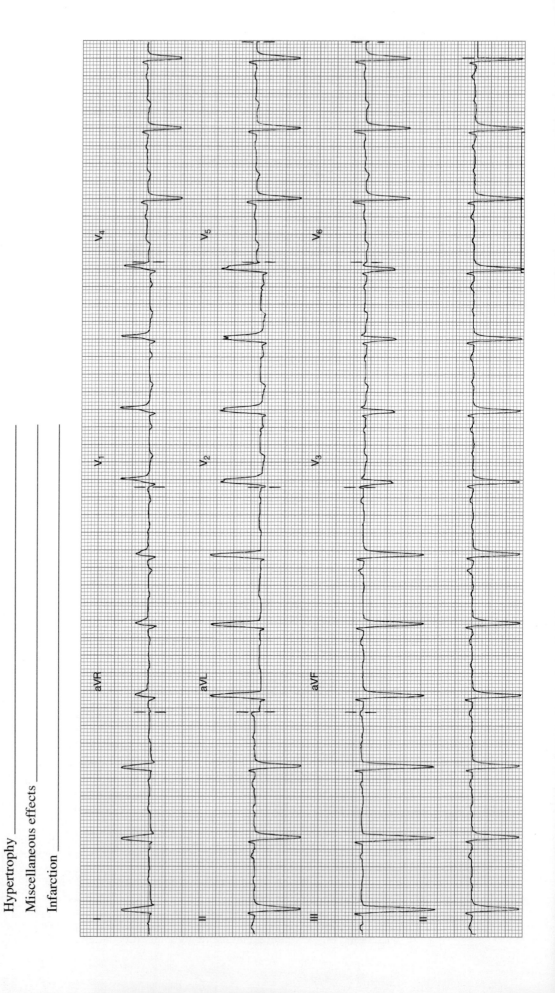

9. Rhythm and rate _____ PR _____ QRS _____ QT _____

Axis _____ BBB/HB _____

Hypertrophy _____

Miscellaneous effects _____

Infarction _____

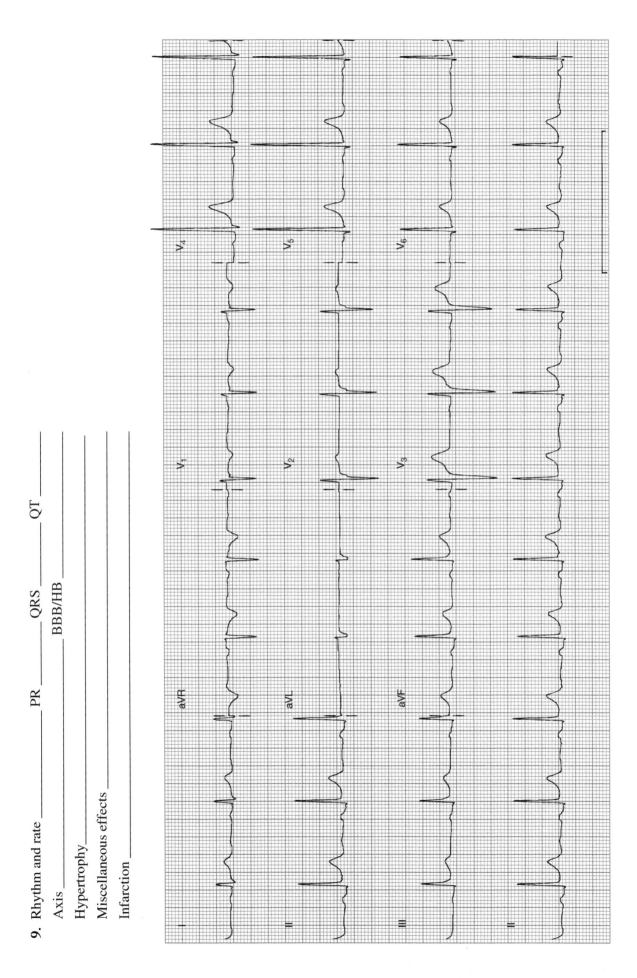

10. Rhythm and rate _____ PR _____ QRS _____ QT _____

Axis _____ BBB/HB _____

Hypertrophy _____

Miscellaneous effects _____

Infarction _____

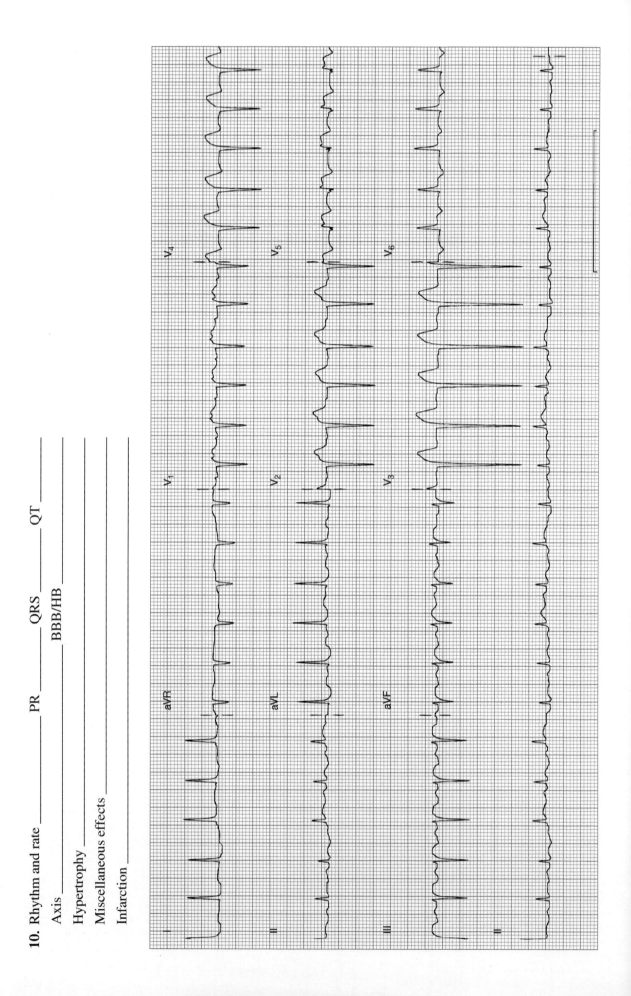

11. Rhythm and rate _____ PR _____ QRS _____ QT _____

Axis _____ BBB/HB _____

Hypertrophy _____

Miscellaneous effects _____

Infarction _____

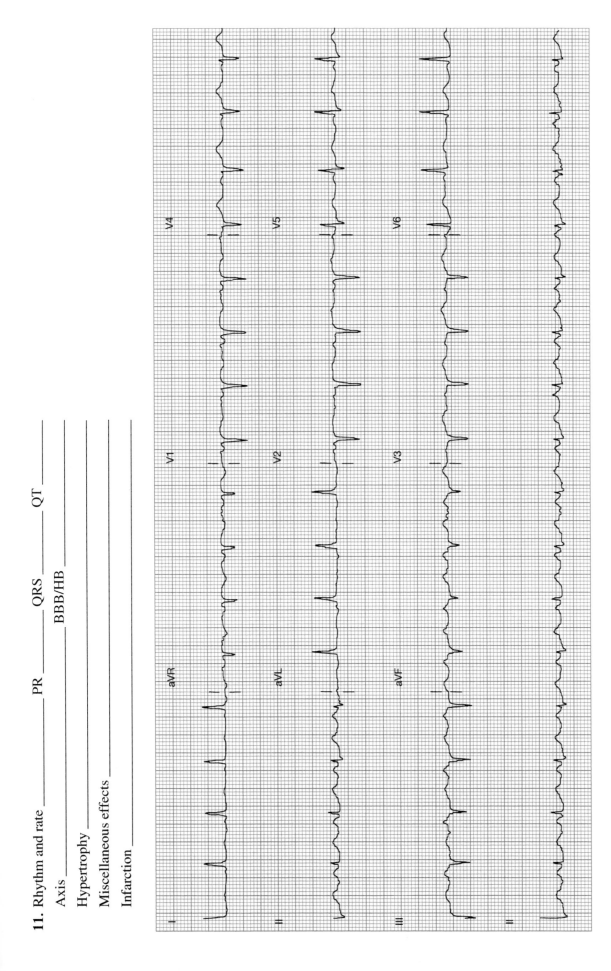

12. Rhythm and rate _____ PR _____ QRS _____ QT _____

Axis _____ BBB/HB _____

Hypertrophy _____

Miscellaneous effects _____

Infarction _____

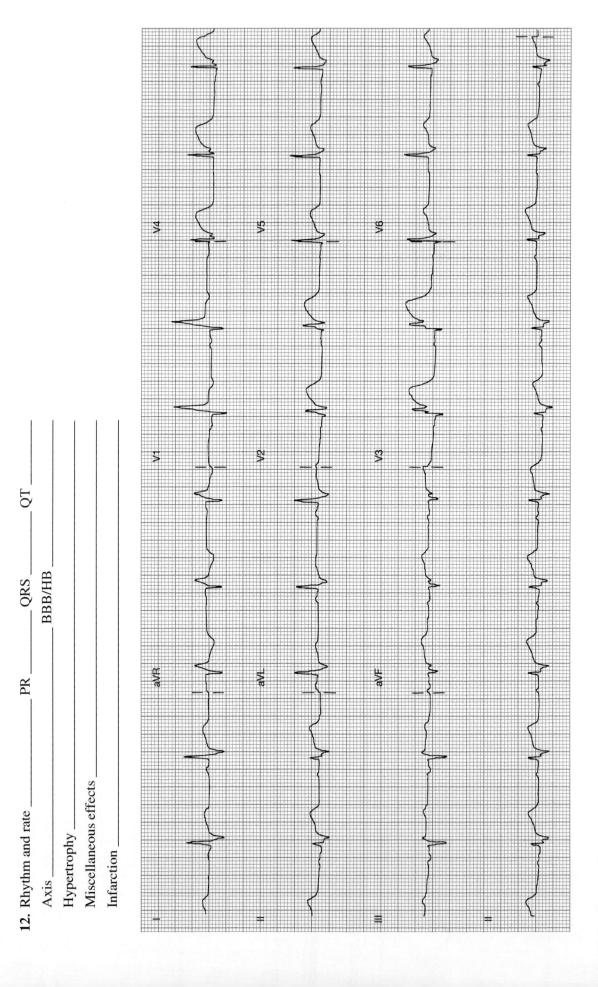

13. Rhythm and rate _____ PR _____ QRS _____ QT _____

Axis _____ BBB/HB _____

Hypertrophy _____

Miscellaneous effects _____

Infarction _____

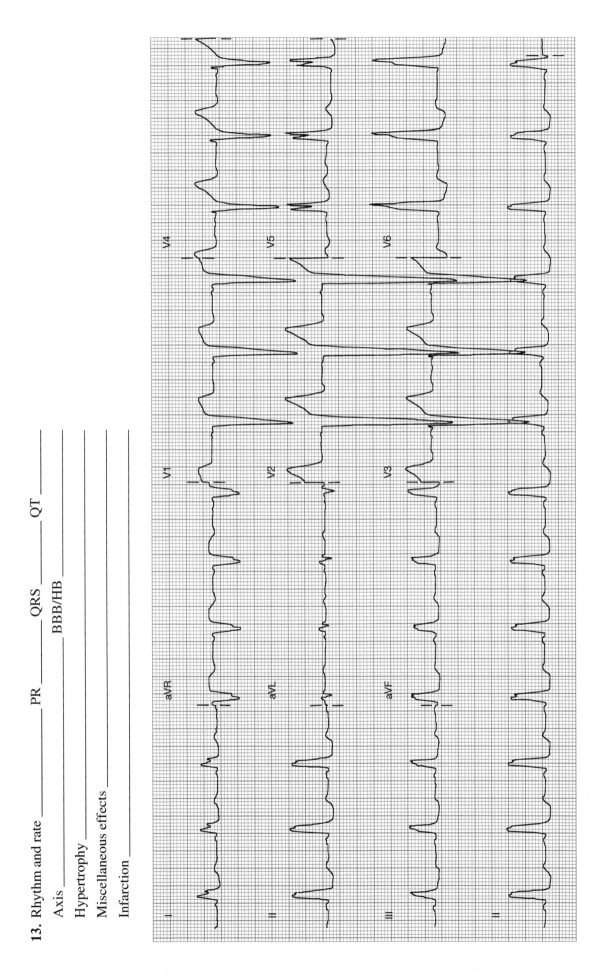

14. Rhythm and rate _____ PR _____ QRS _____ QT _____

Axis _____ BBB/HB _____

Hypertrophy _____

Miscellaneous effects _____

Infarction _____

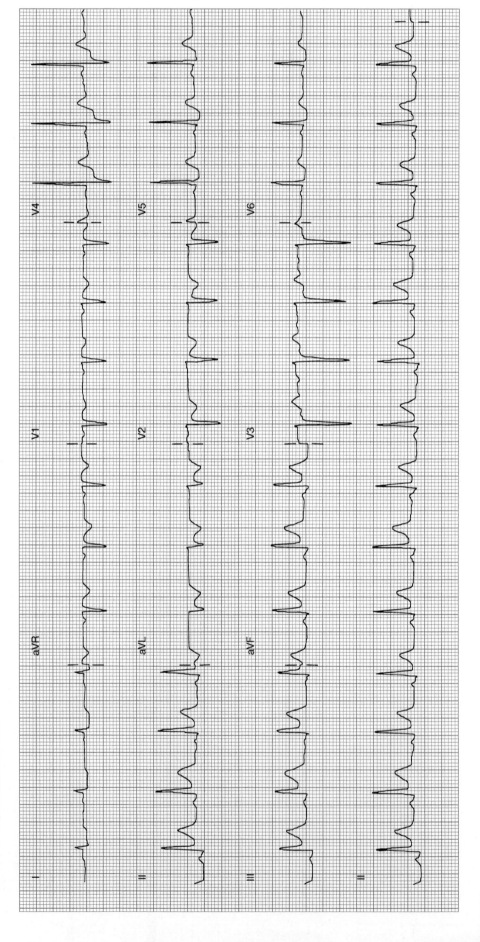

15. Rhythm and rate _____ PR _____ QRS _____ QT _____

Axis _____ BBB/HB _____

Hypertrophy _____

Miscellaneous effects _____

Infarction _____

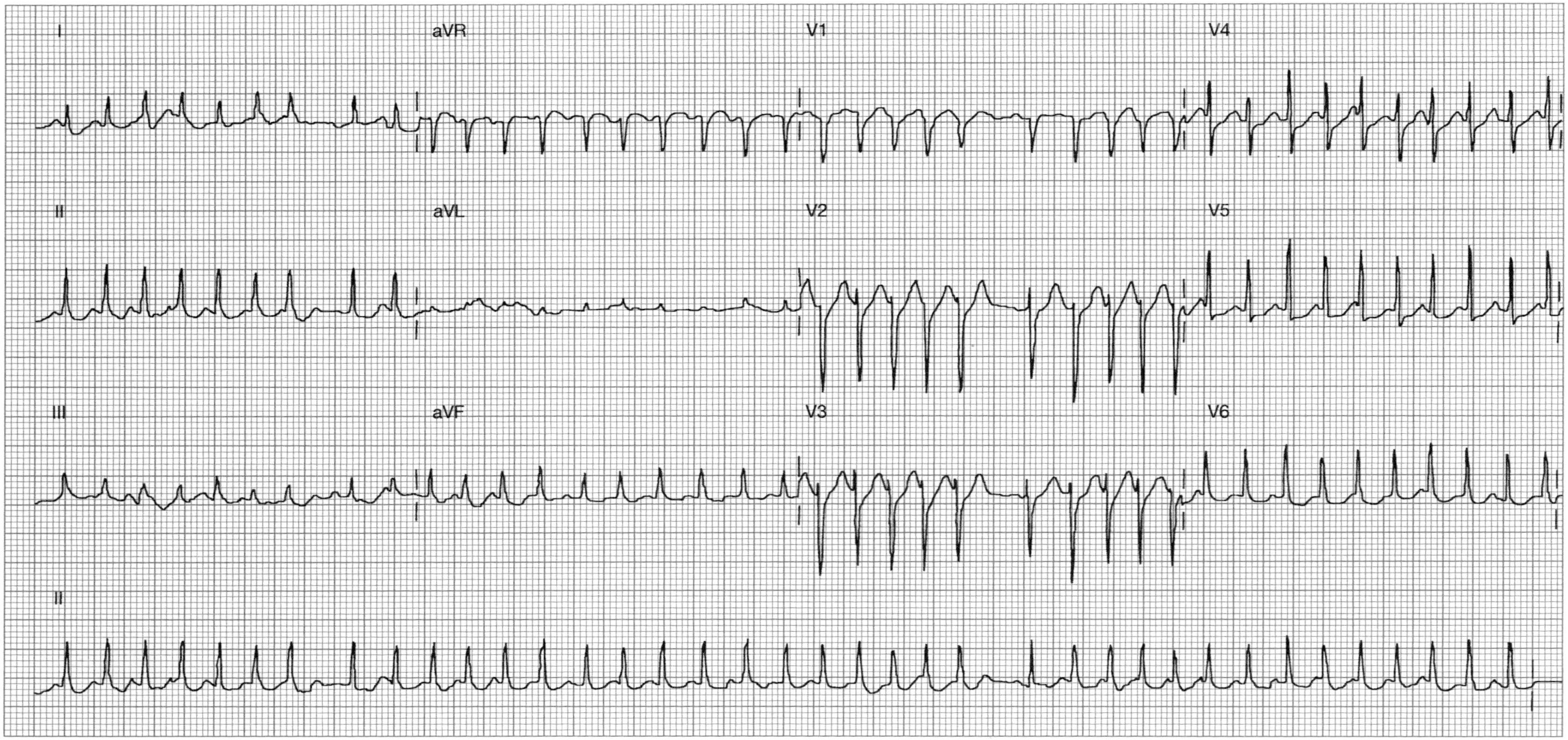

16. Rhythm and rate _____ PR _____ QRS _____ QT _____

Axis _____ BBB/HB _____

Hypertrophy _____

Miscellaneous effects _____

Infarction _____

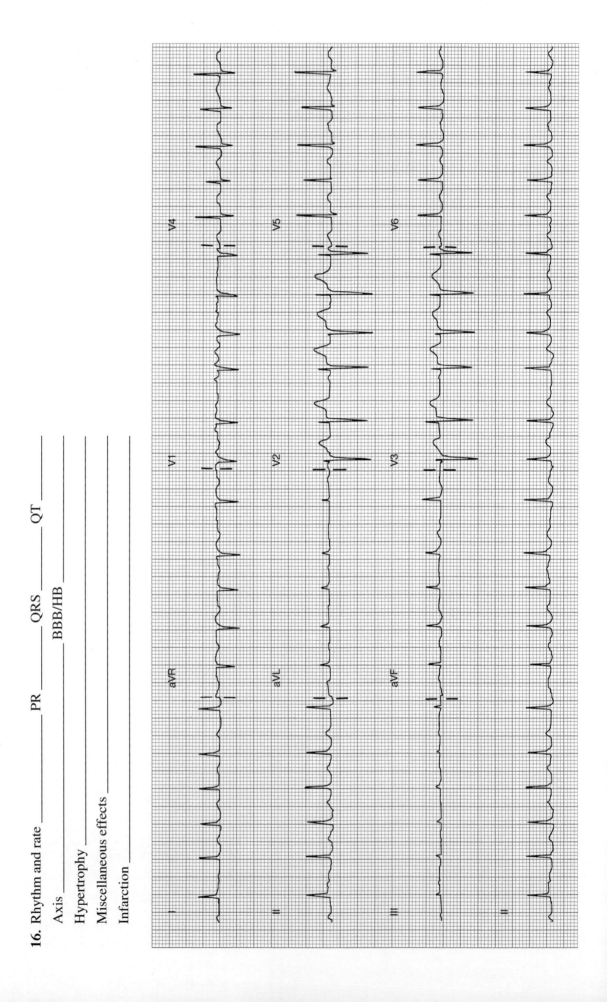

17. Rhythm and rate _____ PR _____ QRS _____ QT _____

Axis _____ BBB/HB _____

Hypertrophy _____

Miscellaneous effects _____

Infarction _____

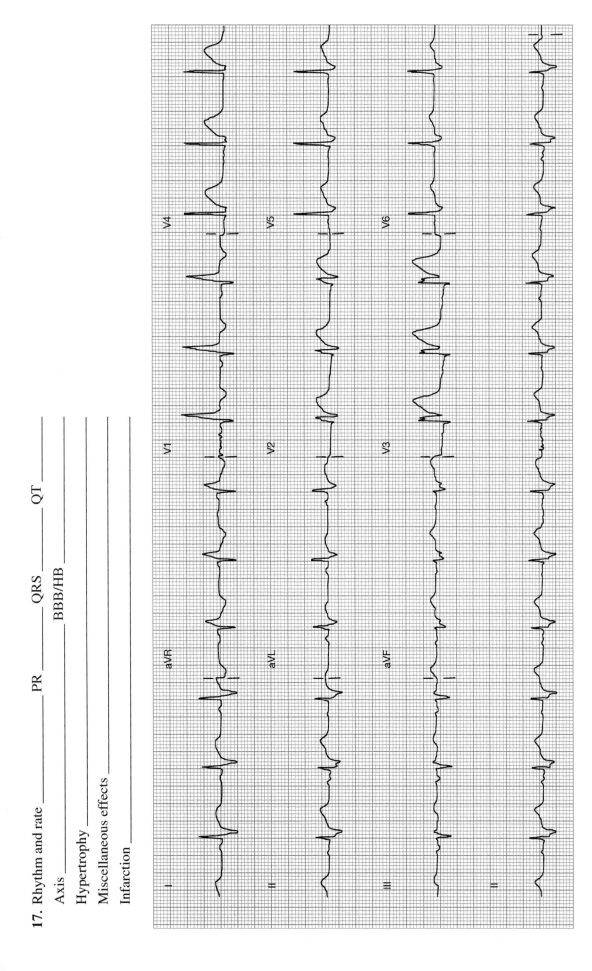

18. Rhythm and rate _____ PR _____ QRS _____ QT _____

Axis _____ BBB/HB _____

Hypertrophy _____

Miscellaneous effects _____

Infarction _____

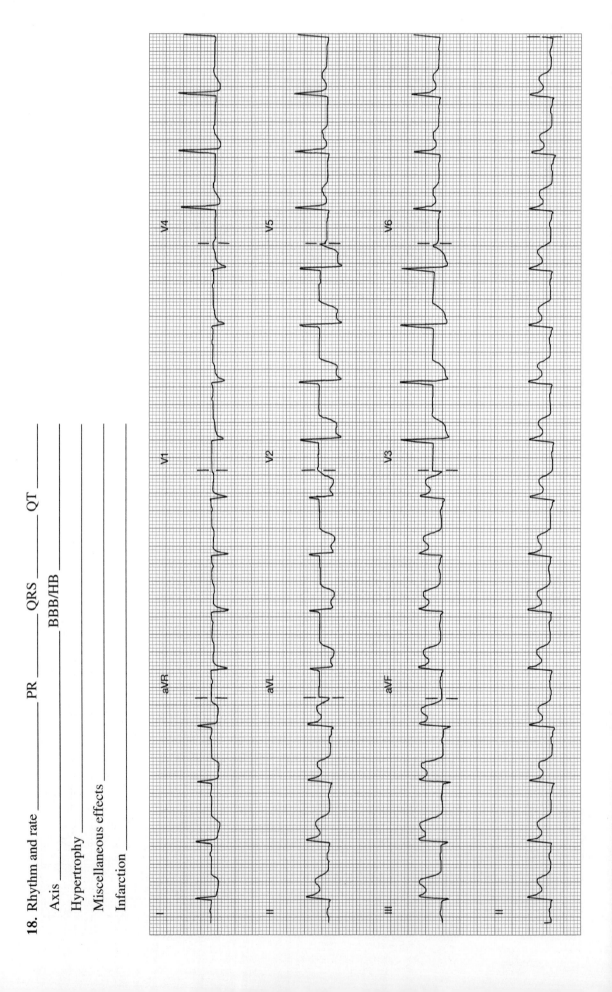

19. Rhythm and rate _____ PR _____ QRS _____ QT _____

Axis _____ BBB/HB _____

Hypertrophy _____

Miscellaneous effects _____

Infarction _____

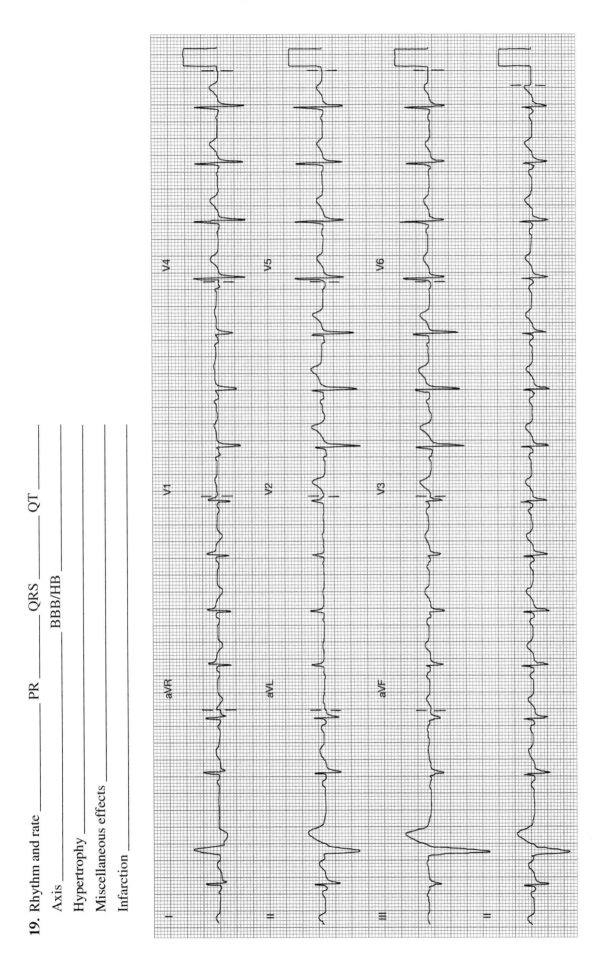

20. Rhythm and rate _____

Axis _____ PR _____ QRS _____ QT _____

Hypertrophy _____ BBB/HB _____

Miscellaneous effects _____

Infarction _____

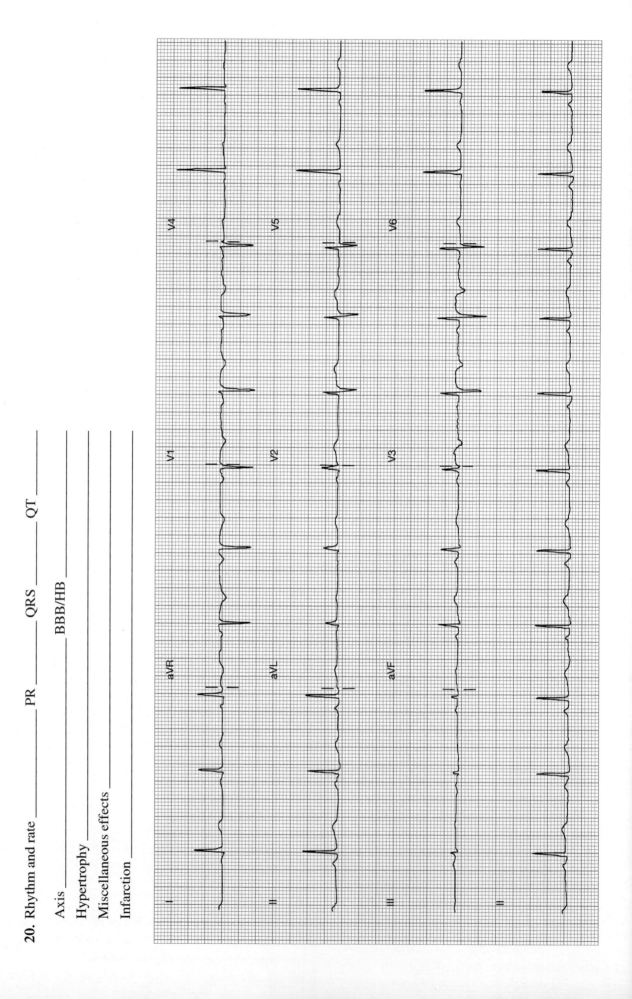

Medications and Electrical Therapy

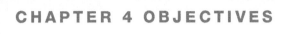

4

CHAPTER 4 OBJECTIVES

Upon completion of this chapter, the student will be able to

- Describe the effect of each class of antiarrhythmic medication on the action potential.
- Give examples of each class of antiarrhythmic medications.
- Describe the effects of digitalis and adenosine on the heart rate.
- Name the emergency medications and describe the mode of action of each.
- Describe the EKG effects of the other covered medications.
- State the primary function of a pacemaker.
- Outline the indications for a pacemaker.
- Name the two components of a permanent pacemaker.
- Describe the types of temporary pacemakers.

- Define the terms *firing, capture,* and *sensing.*
- State what each letter of the pacemaker code means.
- Identify pacemaker rhythms as being either V VI or DDD.
- Identify the different kinds of pacemaker malfunctions.
- Describe the uses and criteria for Cardiac Resynchronization Therapy (CRT).
- Describe when to use cardioversion versus defibrillation.
- Explain the differences between AICD, AED, and monitor/defibrillators.
- Explain the use of therapeutic hypothermia.

What It's All About

The monitor alarm sounded and the ICU nurses shot up from their chairs and ran into Mr. Roman's room. He was in V-tach and had no pulse. "Get the code cart!" yelled the nurse as she pushed the code button to summon help. The code team started chest compressions and began artificial respirations using a special oxygen mask. In no time, the nurses had defibrillated the patient, done two more minutes of CPR, and rechecked the rhythm. It was now a junctional bradycardia with a heart rate of 38. The patient did have a pulse but his blood pressure was very low. "Give atropine and let's get the transcutaneous pacemaker on him at a rate of 60," ordered the physician. The pacemaker did not show capture so the nurse turned up the voltage. That worked. The patient was now showing a beautiful paced rhythm. Within a few minutes, the atropine was kicking in—the patient's heart rate increased and soon he was in sinus rhythm with a heart rate of 83. The pacemaker sensed the patient's inherent rhythm and was no longer firing. When Mr. Roman woke up later and asked what happened, his wife, the physician, and his nurse explained his condition. An angiogram done a few days later showed several narrowed coronary arteries. Mr. Roman had bypass surgery and no further complications.

Introduction

Treatment of arrhythmias can involve medications, electrical shock to the heart, or an electrical stimulus to pace the heart. Let's look at these now.

Medications

Cardiac medications are used to treat arrhythmias or abnormalities in cardiac function. Other medications are used to treat other conditions or diseases, but can have EKG effects. Let's look at the various classifications of medications.

Antiarrhythmics

These medications are used to treat and/or prevent arrhythmias. They all affect the action potential. See Figure 4–1 for the effects of each class on the action potential. There are four classes of antiarrhythmic medications. Let's look at the four classes.

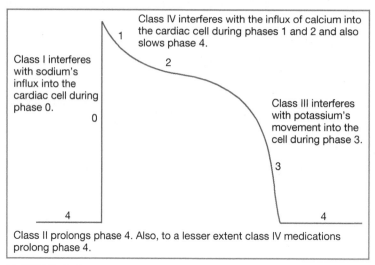

Class IV interferes with the influx of calcium into the cardiac cell during phases 1 and 2 and also slows phase 4.

Class I interferes with sodium's influx into the cardiac cell during phase 0.

Class III interferes with potassium's movement into the cell during phase 3.

Class II prolongs phase 4. Also, to a lesser extent class IV medications prolong phase 4.

FIGURE 4–1

Effects of each class of antiarrhythmic medications on the action potential.

Class I: Sodium Channel Blockers Class I medications block the influx of sodium ions into the cardiac cell during depolarization. This results in decreased excitability of the cardiac cell and decreased myocardial contractility. Class I antiarrhythmic medications affect phase 0 of the action potential. There are three categories of class I antiarrhythmics:

- *Class Ia.* These medications include *quinidine* and *procainamide,* and they cause prolonged QT intervals as well as decreased cardiac contractility. They can also cause hypotension. Quinidine is especially notorious for causing wide T waves. Most class Ia antiarrhythmics can be used to treat supraventricular as well as ventricular arrhythmias. Quinidine is usually given orally. In rare instances it may be given intravenously. Procainamide can be given orally or intravenously. Both these medications have lost favor in current practice, as other meds have proved safer and more therapeutic.
- *Class Ib.* These medications include *lidocaine* and *tocainide,* both of which have a local anesthetic effect. They are used for treatment of ventricular arrhythmias only. They suppress the ventricles' irritability and raise the fibrillatory threshold, making it less likely that the ventricles will fibrillate. Class Ib medications have minimal, if any, effect on conductivity. Lidocaine is given intravenously. Tocainide is given orally.
- *Class Ic.* These medications slow impulse conduction and are useful in treating SVT and ventricular arrhythmias. Unfortunately, they are also prone to causing arrhythmias and are, therefore, used only in life-threatening situations. These medications include *flecainide* and *propafenone,* both of which are given orally.

Class II: Beta-Blockers Beta-blockers slow the heart rate by blocking the sympathetic nervous system's beta-receptors. There are two kinds of beta-receptors: *Beta-1 receptors* increase heart rate, conductivity, and contractility. *Beta-2 receptors* relax smooth muscle in arteries and bronchi. Blocking these receptors decreases or blocks these actions. Beta-blockers decrease the automaticity of the sinus node, slow AV conduction, and slow the process of depolarization. They are used to treat supraventricular tachyarrhythmias (tachycardias that originate above the ventricle). They depress phase 4 of the action potential. Beta-blockers include medications such as *propranolol* and *atenolol*. Propranolol can be given orally or intravenously. Atenolol is given orally. Beta-blockers should be used with caution in patients with asthma or heart failure, as the effects could be life threatening.

Class III: Potassium Channel Blockers Potassium channel blockers interfere with the movement of potassium ions into the cardiac cell during phase 3 of the action potential. They can prolong the PR, QRS, and QT intervals. Class III medications can be used to treat supraventricular and/or ventricular arrhythmias. Medications include *amiodarone,* which is used to treat ventricular and supraventricular tachyarrhythmias, and *ibutilide,* used for supraventricular tachyarrhythmias. Amiodarone can be given orally or intravenously. Ibutilide is given intravenously.

Class IV: Calcium Channel Blockers Calcium channel blockers interfere with the influx of calcium into the cardiac cell during phases 1 and 2 of the action potential and also slow phase 4 of the action potential. Thus, AV conduction is prolonged and contractility decreased. The PR interval will prolong and the heart rate will slow. Calcium blockers are used for supraventricular arrhythmias. Medications include *verapamil* and *diltiazem,* both of which can be given orally or intravenously. Overdose of calcium channel-blockers is treated by administration of calcium.

Let's summarize the antiarrhythmic medications. See Table 4–1.

TABLE 4–1 Antiarrhythmic Medications Summary

Class	Known as	Mode of Action	Examples	Kind of Arrhythmias Treated
I	Sodium channel blockers	Block sodium's influx into the cardiac cell, decrease myocardial excitability and contractility	*Ia.* Quinidine, procainamide *Ib.* Lidocaine, tocainide *Ic.* Flecainide, propafenone	*Ia.* Supraventricular and ventricular *Ib.* Ventricular only *Ic.* Supraventricular and ventricular
II	Beta-blockers	Block the sympathetic nervous system's beta-receptors, slow the heart rate	Propranolol, atenolol	Supraventricular
III	Potassium channel blockers	Decrease potassium's movement into the cardiac cell, prolong PR, QRS, and QT intervals	Amiodarone, ibutilide	Ventricular *or* supraventricular
IV	Calcium channel blockers	Decrease calcium's influx into the cardiac cell, slow AV, conduction, decrease contractility	Verapamil, diltiazem	Supraventricular

Other Antiarrhythmic Medications

There are other antiarrhythmic medications that do not fall into any of the four classes. These include but are not limited to *adenosine,* which is used to treat SVT, and *digitalis,* classified as a cardiac glycoside, which is used to treat heart failure and supraventricular arrhythmias.

Emergency Cardiac Medications

Emergency cardiac medications are used during cardiac arrest or in an arrhythmia-induced life-threatening emergency.

- *Atropine.* Atropine is used to increase the heart rate during bradycardias. It reverses any vagal influence that could slow or stop the heart. It is given intravenously or intraosseous (IO involves a large-bore needle inserted into the marrow of a large bone such as the femur [thigh bone]).
- *Epinephrine.* Epinephrine causes vasoconstriction (narrowing of the arteries), thus increasing the blood pressure, and beta-receptor stimulation, thus restoring the heartbeat and increasing heart rate in cardiac arrest. It is given IV or IO and is used for asystole, V-fib, pulseless V-tach, pulseless electrical activity, and as an infusion for profound bradycardias.
- *Dopamine.* Dopamine increases heart rate and renal blood flow. It can be used as an infusion in bradycardias.
- *Amiodarone.* A class III antiarrhythmic, amiodarone has become the first-line medication for treatment of ventricular fibrillation and pulseless ventricular tachycardia. It can be used to treat supraventricular arrhythmias as well. It is given IV or IO during an emergency and can later be given by mouth to prevent arrhythmia recurrences.
- *Adenosine.* Adenosine is used in emergency situations to convert supraventricular tachycardias back to sinus or to slow the heart rate to a more tolerable level if conversion is not possible. It is given IV and can have the unnerving side effect of causing transient asystole of 6 or 7 seconds before the rhythm converts to sinus.
- *Sodium bicarbonate.* This medication used to be a front-line medication routinely given during cardiac arrest, but its use has fallen out of favor in recent years due to research that has shown it to be potentially damaging if given when not indicated by blood gas studies. Sodium bicarb combats the blood's acidity that develops in the oxygen-deprived setting of cardiac arrest. Combating this acidity can help convert arrhythmias back to normal in a cardiac arrest. Nowadays, sodium bicarb is given most often in prolonged cardiac arrest situations or in those complicated by hyperkalemia. It is given IV.
- *Oxygen.* Although most people do not think of oxygen as a medication, when it is used to treat disease or a medical condition, it is indeed a medication. Oxygen is used to provide the tissues with the oxygen they are lacking. This alone can help convert arrhythmias back to normal. Oxygen can be given by mask, nasal cannula (small prongs in the nose), endotracheal tube (a tube inserted into the trachea by way of the mouth), and tracheotomy (surgically inserting a tube through the neck into the trachea).

Let's summarize the emergency medications. See Table 4–2.

Other Medications with EKG Effects

The following medications are given for non-EKG-related purposes, but they have effects on the heart rhythm or heart rate.

- Diuretics. These are medications given to increase the urine output in patients with heart failure, renal disease, or hypertension. Examples of diuretics include but are not limited to *furosemide, bumetanide, ethacrynic acid,* and *mannitol.* Because diuretics cause increased urination, they can result in dehydration and electrolyte disturbances such as hypokalemia. Hypokalemia, you'll recall, is low

TABLE 4-2 Emergency Medications Summary

Medication	Mode of Action	Indication
Atropine	Increases heart rate	Bradycardias
Epinephrine	Stimulates contractility, increases heart rate and BP	Cardiac arrest, bradycardias
Dopamine	Increases heart rate	Bradycardias
Amiodarone	Helps convert rapid ventricular and supraventricular arhythmias back to sinus	Rapid ventricular arrhythmias, PVCs, supraventricular arrhythmias
Adenosine	Decreases heart rate	Supraventricular tachycardias
Sodium bicarbonate	Decreases blood's acidity	Cardiac arrest with acidosis; hyperkalemia
Oxygen	Increases tissue oxygenation	Symptomatic arrhythmias, cardiac arrest

blood potassium level, and it can cause ventricular irritability and ventricular arrhythmias such as V-tach. Dehydration decreases cardiac output and can result in tachycardias.

- Bronchodilators.   These are medications that dilate narrowed airways in patients with asthma or chronic lung disease. Examples of bronchodilators include *albuterol, levalbuterol, perbuterol, salmeterol,* and *formoterol.* Bronchodilators often cause tachycardia—sometimes with heart rates up to the 140s to 150s. This tachycardia can cause decreased cardiac output, cardiac ischemia, and chest pain.

- Antihypertensives.   These are medications given to treat high blood pressure. They can include diuretics (which we've already discussed), beta-blockers, and vasodilators. Beta-blockers treat hypertension by decreasing the workload of the heart and by dilating arterial walls; however, because of their slowing action on the AV node, they can also result in AV blocks or other kinds of bradycardia. Examples of beta-blockers are *esmolol, propranolol, metoprolol,* and *labetalol*. Vasodilators relax the walls of arteries and/or veins and thereby lower the blood pressure. This can also decrease cardiac output and result in tachycardia. Examples of vasodilators include *hydralazine, nitroglycerin* and *diltiazem.*

- Nitrates.   These are medications given to dilate the coronary arteries and improve coronary blood flow, thus reducing or eliminating chest pain. The typical example is *nitroglycerin tablets.*

- Glaucoma medications.   These are eye drops used to decrease the intraocular (eyeball) pressure. There are many kinds of glaucoma meds, but one kind is a beta-blocker, which as you know can cause bradycardias. An example of beta-blocker eyedrops is *timolol.*

- Erectile dysfunction medications.   This type of medication, such as *sildenafil* and *tadalafil*, can cause a profound drop in blood pressure as well as cardiac ischemia, MI, and tachycardias, especially if these medications are taken by patients who use prescription nitrates such as nitroglycerin for chest pain.

- Tricyclic antidepressants (TCA).   TCAs such as *amitriptyline* and *dosulepin* are used to treat clinical depression. Unfortunately, they are also used with some frequency in suicide attempts by overdose. At toxic levels, TCAs can cause bradycardias including AV blocks, as well as sinus tachycardia, unstable ventricular arrhythmias, asystole, widened QRS, and prolonged PR and QT intervals.

- ***Illegal drugs (cocaine, amphetamines, ecstasy).*** These are used for their "buzz." They have wide-ranging cardiac effects, including, but not limited to, prolonged QT intervals predisposing to torsades de pointes; hypotension, hypertension, tachycardias, AV blocks, myocardial ischemia and/or MI, and coronary artery spasm.

- Thrombolytics. These include *alteplase* and *tenecteplase* and they are used to dissolve the blood clot causing a heart attack or stroke. They can result in bleeding that can increase heart rate. If thrombolytics are successful at aborting a STEMI in progress, the elevated ST segment should return to normal or near-normal.

- Anticoagulants. These are used to prevent blood clots and are routinely used in patients with atrial fibrillation, MI, and other conditions that can predispose patients to blood clots. Because anticoagulants are blood thinners, bleeding can result and lead to tachycardias.

As you can see, although all of these medications/drugs are used for non-EKG-related purposes, they have EKG effects. Always look at *all* your patient's medications to determine if any of them may be causing his or her rhythm or rate disturbances. Also consider that your patient's various medications may be *interacting* and causing rhythm and rate problems. And don't forget to ask about illegal/recreational drugs. Check out Table 4–3.

TABLE 4–3   Other Medications with EKG Effects Summary

Type of Medication	Examples	Used for	Cardiac Effects
Diuretics	Furosemide, bumetanide, mannitol, ethacrynic acid	Heart failure, renal failure, hypertension	Ventricular irritability, ventricular arrhythmias, tachycardias
Bronchodilators	Albuterol, salmeterol, formoterol	Asthma, COPD	Tachycardias, cardiac ischemia, chest pain
Antihypertensives (beta-blockers)	Esmolol, metoprolol, labetolol	Hypertension	Bradycardias, AV blocks, hypotension
Antihypertensives (vasodilators)	Hydralazine, diltiazem, nitroglycerin	Hypertension	Hypotension, tachycardias
Nitrates	Nitroglycerin tablets	Chest pain	Tachycardias, cardiac ischemia or MI
Glaucoma medication	Timolol eyedrops	Glaucoma	Bradycardias
Erectile dysfunction medications	Sildenafil, tadalafil	Erectile dysfunction	Profound hypotension if used when already on nitrates for chest pain; tachycardias, cardiac ischemia and/or MI
Tricyclic antidepressants	Amitriptyline, dosulepin	Clinical depression	Bradycardias including AV blocks, sinus tachycardia, prolonged PR and QT intervals, ventricular arrhythmias, asystole
Illegal drugs	Cocaine, amphetamines, ecstasy	Recreation	Prolonged QT intervals predisposing to torsades de pointes; hypotension, hypertension, tachycardias, AV blocks, myocardial ischemia and/or MI, and coronary artery spasm.
Thrombolytics	Tenecteplase, alteplase	Acute STEMI	Tachycardias secondary to bleeding, ST segment normalization
Anticoagulants	Warfarin	Atrial fibrillation, MI, other conditions	Tachycardias secondary to bleeding

We're about halfway through this chapter. To evaluate your understanding of the material thus far, answer the following questions. If you have trouble with them, review the material again before continuing.

Mrs. Popov, 88 years old, is in SVT with a heart rate of 166. Her blood pressure is dropping, and she's complaining of feeling lightheaded. The physician orders a medication to be

given, and it works, although it did cause a transient spell of asystole before the rhythm converted back to sinus.

1. What was the medication?
2. What other medications could have been given to treat the SVT?

Electrical Therapy

Electrical therapy involves utilizing electrical stimuli to either speed up (or in some cases slow down) the heart rate or to shock the heart out of a dangerous or unstable rhythm. There are two kinds of electrical therapy—artificial pacemakers (traditional and Cardiac Resynchronization Therapy) and cardioversion/defibrillation.

Traditional Artificial Pacemakers

The primary function of an artificial pacemaker is to prevent the heart rate from becoming too slow. Pacemakers provide an electrical stimulus when the heart is unable to generate its own or when its own is too slow to provide adequate cardiac output. You'll recall from Chapter 10 that pacemakers can pace the atrium, the ventricle, or both.

Another use for pacemakers is antitachycardia pacing (also called overdrive pacing). This special programming function on some pacemakers allows the pacemaker to interrupt a tachycardia by interjecting a series of paced beats in the middle of the tachycardia, thus interrupting the rapid circuit and allowing the sinus node to resume control. On other pacemakers without the antitachycardia pacing function, the physician can simply stand at the patient's bedside and increase the pacemaker's heart rate until it exceeds the tachycardia. This puts the pacemaker in control and abolishes the tachycardia. The pacemaker's heart rate can then be decreased back down to a normal rate.

> **Quick Tip**
>
> *Pacemakers do not force the heart to beat.* They simply send out an electrical signal, just as the heart's normal pacemakers do. If the heart is healthy enough, it should respond to that stimulus by depolarizing.

Indications

Indications for a pacemaker may include the following:

- Symptomatic sinus bradycardia
- Junctional rhythms
- Idioventricular rhythm
- Dying heart
- Asystole
- 2:1 AV block
- Mobitz II second-degree AV block
- Third degree AV block
- Antitachycardia pacing

Permanent Versus Temporary Pacemakers

A permanent pacemaker is inserted when the arrhythmia that necessitates it is thought to be permanent. It has two components—a *pulse generator* (a battery pack), inserted surgically into a pocket made just under the right or left clavicle, and a *pacing catheter,* which is inserted via the subclavian vein into the superior vena cava and down into the right atrium and/or ventricle. Permanent pacemaker batteries are made of lithium and usually last between 5 and 15 years. See Figure 4–2.

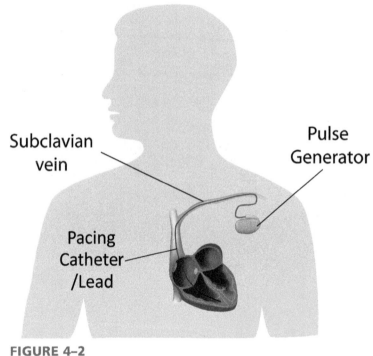

FIGURE 4–2

Pulse generator and pacing catheter of a permanent pacemaker (Alila Medical Media/Shutterstock).

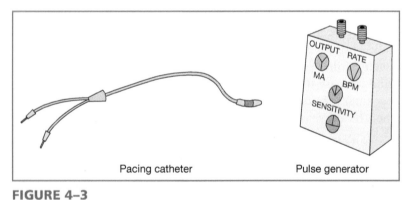

FIGURE 4–3

Transvenous pacemaker components.

Temporary pacemakers are used to help the patient "get over the hump" after an MI or other problem temporarily causes symptomatic bradycardia. Temporary pacemakers come in various types, the two most common being the transvenous, in which a pacing catheter is inserted into a large vein and threaded into the right atrium and down into the right ventricle, and the transcutaneous, which involves large pacing electrodes attached to the chest and back that pace the heart through the chest wall. Both of these temporary pacer methods require a pulse generator at the patient's bedside. See Figures 4–3 and 4–4.

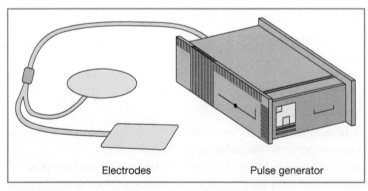

FIGURE 4–4

Transcutaneous pacemaker components.

Pacemaker Terminology

Firing refers to the pacemaker's generation of an electrical stimulus. It is noted on the EKG by the presence of a *pacemaker spike*.

Capture refers to the presence of a P wave or a QRS complex (or both) after the pacemaker spike. This indicates that the tissue in the chamber being paced has depolarized. The pacemaker is then said to have "captured" that chamber. Paced QRS complexes are wide and bizarre and resemble PVCs.

Sensing refers to the pacemaker's ability to recognize the patient's own intrinsic rhythm or beats in order to decide if it needs to fire. Most pacemakers function on a *demand mode,* meaning they fire only when needed (only on demand).

Three-Letter Pacemaker Code

Pacemakers are referred to by a three-letter code:

- The first letter refers to the *chamber paced*.
  V = ventricle
  A = atrium
  D = dual (atrium and ventricle)
  O = none
- The second letter refers to the *chamber sensed*.
  V = ventricle
  A = atrium
  D = dual (atrium and ventricle)
  O = none
- The third letter refers to the *response to sensed events*.
  I = inhibited (pacemaker watches and waits, does not pace until needed)
  T = triggered (pacemaker sends out a signal in response to a sensed event)
  D = dual (inhibited and triggered)
  O = none

Let's look at the codes in a little more depth. What would a VOO pacemaker do, for example? The first letter refers to the chamber paced, so the VOO paces the ventricle. The second letter refers to the chamber sensed, so it senses nothing. Because it senses nothing, it obviously can't have a response to sensed events, so the last letter has to be O also. A VOO pacemaker is called a fixed-rate pacemaker because it will fire at its programmed rate regardless of the patient's own rate at the time. This is dangerous, because if the pacemaker spike hits on top of the T wave of the patient's own (intrinsic) beats, it could cause V-tach or V-fib. Fixed-rate pacemakers are not used today. All pacemakers in use today are *demand pacemakers*. They have a sensor that tells the pacemaker when to fire.

VVI Pacemakers

The most common kinds of pacemakers in use today are the VVI and the DDD. The VVI pacemaker, also known as a ventricular demand pacemaker, was at one time the most commonly used permanent pacer. It's now in second place. The VVI pacer consists of a catheter with both pacing and sensing capabilities and is inserted into the right ventricle. See Figure 4–5.

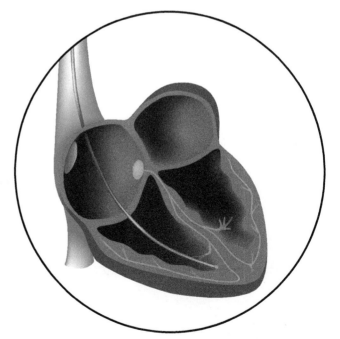

FIGURE 4–5

VVI pacemaker inserted into the right ventricle (Alila Medical Media/ Shutterstock).

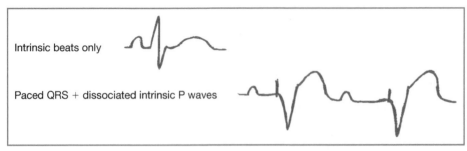

Intrinsic beats only

Paced QRS + dissociated intrinsic P waves

FIGURE 4–6

VVI pacemaker options.

The VVI pacemaker paces the ventricle, providing a spike and then a wide QRS complex. It senses the ventricle, so it looks for intrinsic QRS complexes to determine if it needs to fire. Let's say the patient is in a sinus rhythm with a heart rate of 80 and the pacemaker is set at a rate of 60. The sensor would "see" the patient's own QRS complexes and realize it does not need to fire. It will be inhibited. If the patient's heart rate falls to a rate below the pacemaker's preset heart rate, the pacer will see that the QRS complexes are not at a fast enough rate, so it will fire and pace the heart. As with your own conduction system, whichever is the fastest pacemaker is the one in control. Because the VVI pacer senses only intrinsic QRS complexes, it ignores the P waves. Therefore, *there will be no relationship between P waves and paced QRS complexes.*

VVI pacemakers provide two options:

- *Intrinsic beats only.*   The pacemaker does not pace because it doesn't need to. The rhythm is fast enough, so the pacemaker is inhibited. There will be no pacemaker spikes. The rhythm is produced completely by the patient.
- *Paced QRS, dissociated intrinsic P waves.*   The pacemaker senses and paces only the ventricle. There will be pacemaker spikes preceding only the QRS complexes. Intrinsic P waves, if present, will be ignored by the pacemaker. See Figure 4–6.

DDD Pacemakers

The DDD pacemaker is the most modern and the most physiologic. It is known as a universal pacemaker and is now the most commonly inserted permanent pacemaker. It paces and senses both atrium and ventricle. See Figure 4–7.

The DDD pacemaker senses intrinsic atrial activity and takes advantage of the patient's own P waves. If the DDD pacemaker senses the patient's P waves within its preset rate, it will not need to give another P wave, so its atrial pacer will be inhibited. The ventricle, however, will then be triggered to give a QRS if the patient does not have his or her own QRS in the preset length of time after the P wave. *DDD pacemakers provide a constant relationship between P waves and QRS complexes.* If the pacemaker senses intrinsic P waves and QRS complexes within the appropriate time interval, it will be inhibited; it will just watch and wait until it's needed. If there are no Ps or QRS complexes in the preset time interval, the pacemaker will pace both chambers, providing a paced P and a paced QRS. Basically, the DDD provides whatever the patient cannot do on his or her own.

DDD pacemakers are usually rate-responsive, meaning that they will provide a paced QRS to follow the patient's intrinsic P waves within preset heart rate limits. These limits are usually 60 to 125. Within this range, the DDD pacemaker will provide a paced QRS for every intrinsic P wave. Below these limits, the pacemaker will provide paced P waves also, as the intrinsic atrial rate is too slow. Above these limits, the DDD pacemaker will

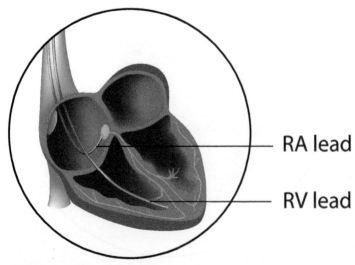

RA lead

RV lead

FIGURE 4–7

DDD pacemaker and sensor wires in right atrium and ventricle (Alila Medical Media/Shutterstock).

not provide a paced QRS for each intrinsic P wave because that would result in a tachycardia dangerous to the patient.

Let's break that down a bit. Say the patient has an underlying third-degree AV block, which means a lot of P waves compared to QRS complexes. If the atrial rate (the rate of the P waves, you'll recall) is between 60 and 125, the DDD pacemaker will "track the P waves." This means the pacemaker will provide a paced QRS complex as needed to follow each intrinsic P wave. It will not provide paced P waves, because it won't need to; the patient has his or her own Ps at a fast enough rate.

If the atrial rate drops below 60, the rate of the P waves is too slow; the DDD pacemaker will then provide paced P waves as well as QRS complexes as needed to keep the heart rate within the range of 60 to 125.

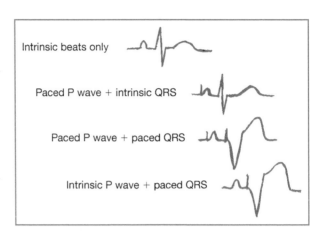

FIGURE 4–8

DDD pacemaker options.

If the atrial rate exceeds 125, the P waves are now too fast; the DDD pacemaker will ignore some of those P waves and track others. Therefore, there may be paced QRS complexes after only every second or third intrinsic P wave, and so forth. Why does it do this? If the atrial rate is faster than 125, and the pacemaker provides a paced QRS after each P wave, the patient ends up with a heart rate of 125. That may be so fast that cardiac output drops. If the atrial rate exceeds the upper limit, the pacemaker senses the atrial rate and decides to obey only some, rather than all, of the intrinsic P waves.

DDD pacemakers provide four options:

- *Intrinsic beats only.* The pacemaker does not fire because it does not need to. The intrinsic rate is fast enough. There will be no pacemaker spikes.
- *Paced P wave, intrinsic QRS.* The pacemaker paces the atrium, providing a pacemaker spike and a paced P wave. Following this, the patient's own QRS occurs. There is therefore a spike only before the P wave.
- *Paced P wave, paced QRS.* The pacemaker paces both chambers, providing a spike before the P wave and a spike before the QRS.
- *Intrinsic P wave, paced QRS.* The patient has his or her own P waves, so the pacemaker tracks them and provides a paced QRS to follow. There is a pacemaker spike only before the QRS. See Figure 4–8.

DDD Versus VVI Practice

On the following strips, tell whether the pacemaker is DDD or VVI (or undeterminable).

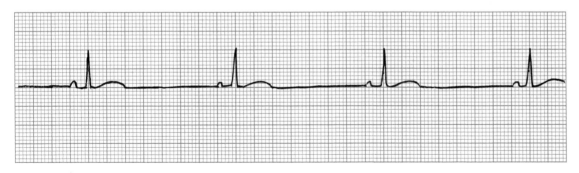

1. _____

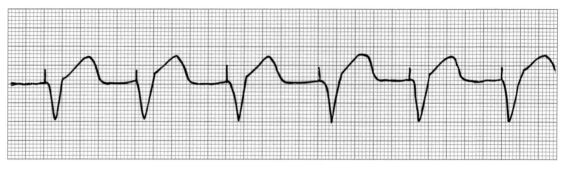

2. _____

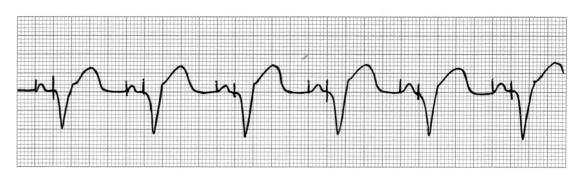

3. _____

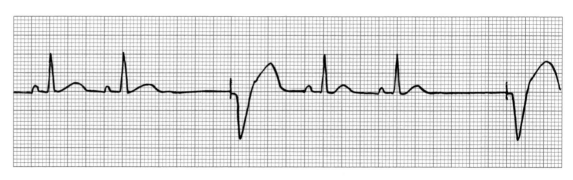

4. _____

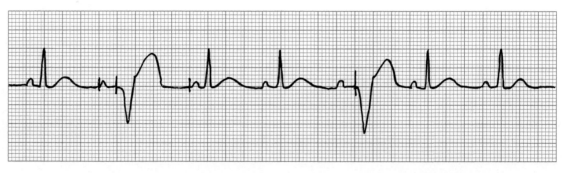

5. _____

Pacemaker Malfunctions

Like any gadget, pacemakers sometimes malfunction. The typical malfunctions include:

- *Failure to Fire.* Here the pacemaker fails to send out its electrical stimulus when it should. This can mean the pacemaker battery is dead or the connecting wires are interrupted. Or it can mean the pacemaker has oversensed something like extraneous muscle artifact and thinks it's not supposed to fire. Failure to fire is evidenced by the lack of pacemaker spikes where they should have been. It usually results in a pause. Figure 4–9 is an example of failure to fire.

   In Figure 4–9, assume the patient's pacemaker rate is set at 60. There are no pacemaker spikes anywhere. The rhythm is a slow sinus bradycardia with a heart rate of about 28. The pacemaker should have prevented the heart rate from going this slowly, but it didn't fire.

- *Loss of Capture.* There is no P or QRS after the pacemaker spike in loss of capture. This is often simply a matter of turning up the pacemaker's voltage so that it sends out more "juice" to tell the heart what to do. Maybe the signal it sent out was too weak to get a response from the chamber. Another possibility is that the pacing catheter has lost contact with the wall of the chamber it is in and cannot cause depolarization. That could be corrected by a simple position change of the patient, or it could necessitate minor surgery to adjust the catheter placement. Loss of capture can also occur when the heart is too damaged to respond to the pacer's stimulus. See Figure 4–10 for an example of loss of capture.

   Figure 4–10 shows asystole with pacemaker spikes but no Ps or QRS complexes after the spikes. The pacemaker has fired, as evidenced by the spikes, but it has not captured the chamber it is in.

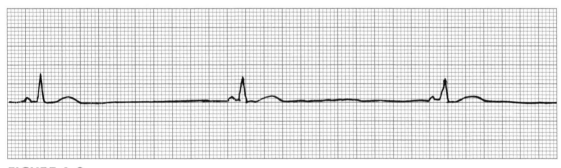

FIGURE 4–9

Failure to fire.

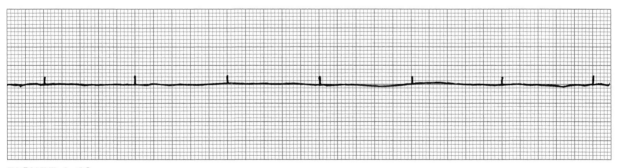

FIGURE 4–10

Loss of capture.

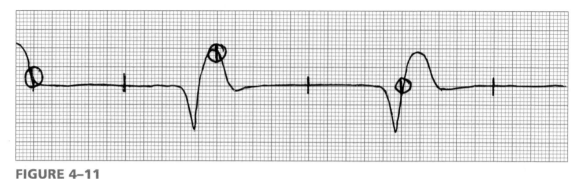

FIGURE 4–11

Undersensing.

- *Undersensing.*   Here the pacemaker fires too soon after an intrinsic beat, often resulting in pacemaker spikes where they shouldn't have been, such as in a T wave, an ST segment, or right on top of another QRS. This happens when the pacemaker just doesn't see that other beat. The pacemaker's sensor needs adjusting. Another possibility is a fractured sensing wire or battery failure. In Figure 4–11 we have undersensing.

  In Figure 4–11, note the spikes at times when the pacer should not have fired. How do you detect undersensing? Look at the distance between two consecutive pacemaker spikes. That's the normal pacing interval, which will correspond to a certain paced heart rate. *There should be exactly that same distance between the patient's own intrinsic beats and the next paced beat.* If the distance is less than that, there is undersensing. In Figure 4–11, the circled pacemaker spikes indicate undersensing.

  But this strip also shows another malfunction. Do you know what it is? Look it over carefully before continuing.

  There is loss of capture in addition to the undersensing. All the uncircled spikes plus the first circled one did not result in a P wave or QRS complex at a time when they should have. The second and third circled spikes would not be considered loss of capture even though they also don't result in a P or QRS. Why? Remember the refractory periods? From the beginning of the QRS to the upstroke of the T wave is the absolute refractory period. A spike that occurs during that time cannot possibly capture. That's not a pacemaker malfunction; it's just physiology.

  For a summary of pacemaker malfunctions, see Table 4–4.

TABLE 4–4   Pacemaker Malfunctions Summary

Pacemaker Malfunctions	EKG Evidence
Failure to fire	Lack of pacemaker spikes where they should have been. Usually results in a pause.
Loss of capture	Pacemaker spikes not followed by P waves or QRS complexes.
Undersensing	Paced beats or spikes too close to previous beats. Often results in spikes inside T waves, ST segments, or QRS complexes.

Pacemaker Malfunctions Practice

On the strips that follow, indicate the pacer malfunction(s), if any.

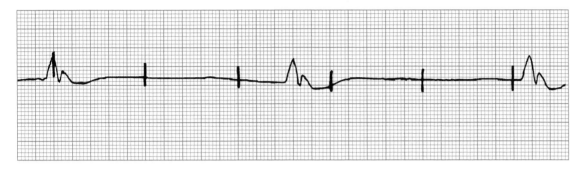

Situation: This patient passed out at home. The paramedics found him with a barely palpable, very slow pulse. His VVI pacemaker is set at 60.

1. _____

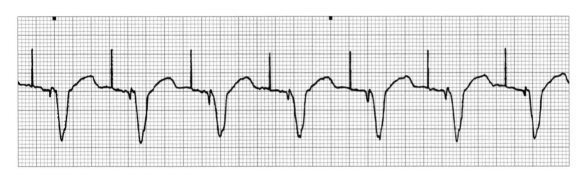

Situation: This patient had a DDD pacemaker inserted 3 years ago and now appears in the ER complaining of sudden onset of dizziness and syncope. The pacemaker rate is set at 68.

2. _____

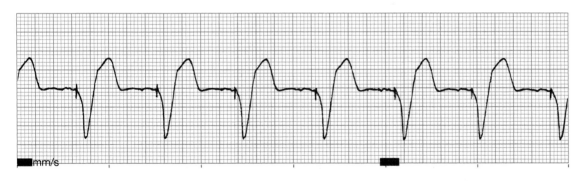

Situation: This patient has a DDD pacemaker set at 72. She is seen in her doctor's office for a routine checkup. She feels fine.

3. _____

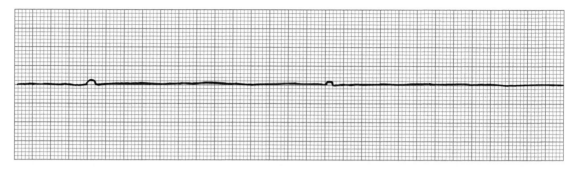

Situation: This patient is seen in the ER in cardiac arrest. His DDD pacemaker is set at 70.

4. _____

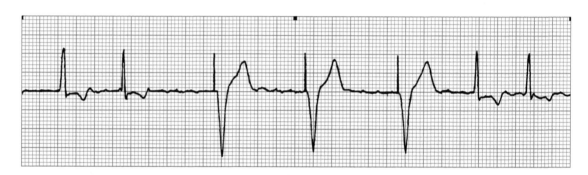

Situation: This patient had a VVI pacemaker inserted recently because of slow atrial fibrillation. It's set at 60. She feels fine.

5. _____

The Problem with Traditional Pacemakers

As beneficial as they are, the pacemakers we've reviewed thus far have one big problem—they cause dyssynchrony (abnormal timing) between the right and left atria or between the right and left ventricles. In the normal heart, the atria are stimulated simultaneously and contract as a unit to empty their blood into the ventricles, then the ventricles are stimulated simultaneously and contract together to pump the blood out to the lungs and the systemic circulation. With a traditional pacemaker, instead of both atria or both ventricles contracting simultaneously, they're contracting sequentially (one after the other). *Traditional pacemakers pace only the right atrium or right ventricle or both—not the left side. If one chamber is stimulated before the other, it contracts before the other.* This dyssynchrony decreases ventricular filling and can decrease cardiac output—not a good thing if a patient is in congestive heart failure (CHF) and needs both ventricles to work together to maximize pumping efficiency.

Cardiac Resynchronization Therapy (CRT) was developed to help CHF patients obtain/maintain an adequate cardiac output.

Cardiac Resynchronization Therapy

Cardiac Resynchronization Therapy (CRT) involves the use of a biventricular pacemaker a type of pacemaker in which there are pacing electrodes in the right atrium and *both ventricles*. See Figure 4–12. Because both ventricles are stimulated simultaneously, they will contract simultaneously, thus improving cardiac output. There are strict criteria for implantation of CRT. The patient must be symptomatic with:

- Severe heart failure (left ventricular ejection fraction (EF) less than 35%). Normal EF (the percentage of blood pumped out by the left ventricle with each beat) is 55%–70%.
- Wide QRS (<0.13 secs) with LBBB.
- Sinus rhythm.

For the appropriately selected CHF patient, CRT can increase the ejection fraction by about 10%, decrease the size of the bloated left ventricle, decrease the QRS interval toward a more normal range, and increase the quality of life.

Let's move on now to other kinds of electrical therapy: electrical cardioversion and defibrillation.

Electrical Cardioversion

The word cardioversion means changing the heart. Electrical cardioversion involves a small electrical shock to the heart, usually performed to convert supraventricular tachycardias back to sinus, but it can also be used for ventricular tachycardia, provided the patient has a pulse. (Pulseless V-tach requires defibrillation, not cardioversion.) The goal here is to interrupt an abnormal electrical circuit within the heart that is allowing an arrhythmia to continue. Electrical cardioversion is performed using a defibrillator that can be set to "synchronous" mode. *Synchronizing is what differentiates cardioversion from defibrillation.* Once the synchronizer button is activated on the defibrillator, the machine delays delivery of the shock until it has synchronized with the patient's QRS complexes. The shock must be delivered at a critical point in the cardiac cycle. *If a shock is delivered at the wrong point in the cardiac cycle, it can put the patient into ventricular fibrillation*—not a good thing if the patient was just in SVT. Perhaps the most critical thing to know about cardioversion is *when not to use it*: Do not try to cardiovert V-fib— this rhythm requires defibrillation. *Turn the synchronizer button off when defibrillating or the shock will not be delivered!*

Defibrillation

Defibrillation differs from cardioversion in that the shock is delivered immediately upon pressing the button. There is no synchronizing in defibrillation. And the electrical current delivered tends to be much larger, causing the entire myocardium to depolarize at once. This interrupts the abnormal rhythm and causes a brief asystole, after which the heart's normal automaticity should cause it to restart with normal conduction. *Defibrillation is the treatment for ventricular fibrillation and pulseless ventricular tachycardia.* There are several kinds of defibrillators: the monitor/defibrillator used in hospitals, AICDs (automated implantable cardioverter-defibrillators), and AEDs (automated external defibrillators). See Figure 4–13 for photos of each. Let's look at these now:

- *Monitor/defibrillator. Is a combination of a cardiac monitor with a 3- or 5-lead cable plus a cardioverter-defibrillator.* It is attached to the patient, and then health care personnel analyze the rhythm and activate the buttons to either cardiovert or

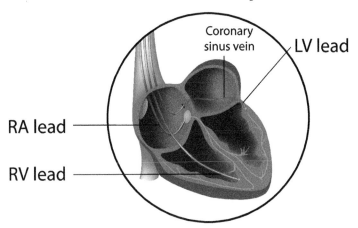

Biventricular / CRT

FIGURE 4–12

Biventricular pacemaker and sensor wires in right atrium, right ventricle, and left ventricle (Alila Medical Media/Shutterstock).

Quick Tip

If the rhythm is *V-fib* you must *defib*!

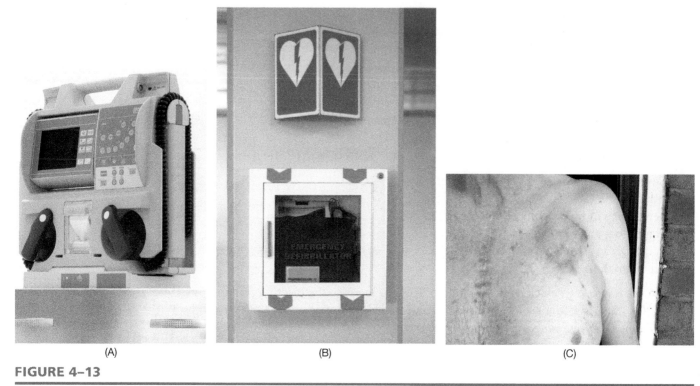

(A)   (B)   (C)

FIGURE 4–13

(A) Monitor-defibrillator (Beerkoff/Shutterstock), **(B) AED** (Eric Gevaert/Shutterstock), **and (C) AICD in patient's left chest** (© Michael F. O'Keefe).

defibrillate the patient. Use of this device requires knowledge of rhythms and their appropriate treatment by the user. Defibrillators come in *monophasic* and *biphasic* types. They deliver their energy/shock in different doses, so it's important to know which type defibrillator is used at your facility.

■ *AICD.*   *Is an implanted device that is programmed to analyze abnormal rhythms and deliver a small internal electrical shock to abort an abnormal rhythm such as V-tach or V-fib.* It is completely contained within the body. The AICD also has a pacemaker that allows it to pace the heart if the shock causes asystole. Antitachycardia pacing is also an option with AICDs.

■ *AED.*   *Is a defibrillator meant for use by the lay public.* It can be found in airports, shopping malls, and on airplanes. Extremely simple to use, the device is attached to the patient and automatically analyzes the rhythm. It can then either tell the rescuer what to do (as in "push the button to defibrillate") or do everything automatically without rescuer intervention. In either case, the AED requires no medical or technical knowledge by the rescuer. The machine, once plugged in, tells the rescuer step by step what to do next.

So what happens to our cardiac arrest patient who has a return of spontaneous circulation (ROSC) after we've defibrillated him or her and given our emergency medications? Let's talk a moment about therapeutic hypothermia.

Therapeutic Hypothermia

Therapeutic hypothermia (TH) involves cooling the post–cardiac arrest patient's body temperature down to about 90 to 93 degrees Fahrenheit in order to reduce the risk of ischemic damage (particularly brain damage) caused by the period of decreased or absent blood flow. It has long been known that lower body temperatures decrease the body's metabolic demands. Research has shown that post–cardiac arrest hypothermia protects/preserves brain function and can help the patient achieve a better outcome.

As an example, let's look at a man who suffers a cardiac arrest at a football game. Paramedics successfully resuscitate the man, who then regains a spontaneous pulse but remains unconscious. (This is an important distinction—TH is not done on conscious patients). Paramedics rush the patient to the closest ER where TH is started. There are several methods of commencing TH, but they typically involve either chilled water blankets or gel pads in contact with the patient's skin, and/or with iced saline fluids IV through a large central vein. Hypothermia is maintained for about 12 to 24 hours and then gradual rewarming is begun.

During the cool-down phase, the PR, QRS, and QT intervals can prolong and there is increased risk for atrial and ventricular arrhythmias. Sinus tachycardia is common at the start of TH, but this usually slows to sinus bradycardia as cooling continues. Hypokalemia is common during cool-down, often necessitating potassium replacement.

The rewarming period is the most dangerous, with electrolyte disturbances (particularly hyperkalemia) very common. Watch for tall pointy T waves and widening QRS complexes.

Cardiac medications and electrical therapy are being constantly updated and improved, and therapeutic hypothermia can help maximize your patients' chance of a good post–cardiac arrest outcome. Keeping up with these advances is critical in caring for your patients.

chapter four notes TO SUM IT ALL UP . . .

- **Classes of antiarrhythmic medications:**
  - *I—Sodium channel blockers*—Decrease myocardial contractility and excitability
    - Ia—Causes prolonged QT interval, decreases contractility, lowers blood pressure
    - Ib—Used for ventricular arrhythmias only
    - Ic—decreases impulse conduction
  - *II—Beta-blockers:*—Decrease sinus node automaticity, slow AV conduction, decrease heart rate
  - *III—Potassium channel blockers:*—Prolong PR, QRS, and QT intervals
  - *IV—Calcium channel blockers:*—Slow AV conduction, decrease contractility, increase PR interval, slow heart rate

- **Emergency cardiac medications:**
  - *Atropine*—Treats bradycardias—speeds up heart rate
  - *Epinephrine*—Treats bradycardias, asystole, V-fib, pulseless V-tach, PEA—increases heart rate and blood pressure
  - *Dopamine*—Used as an infusion for bradycardias—increases heart rate and blood pressure
  - *Amiodarone*—Treats supraventricular and ventricular arrhythmias—helps abolish those rhythms
  - *Adenosine*—Treats SVT—can cause brief asystole before rhythm converts back to sinus
  - *Sodium bicarbonate*—Treats acidosis—used when indicated by blood gas studies
  - *Oxygen*—Used in all emergencies—increases tissue oxygenation and can combat arrhythmias

- **Other medications with EKG effects:**
  - *Diuretics*—Used to increase urine output—can cause dehydration and lead to electrolyte disturbances that can in turn cause ventricular irritability
  - *Bronchodilators*—Used to open narrowed air passages in patients with asthma or chronic lung disease—can cause tachycardias
  - *Antihypertensive medications*—Used to treat hypertension—can cause tachycardias or bradycardias, AV blocks, hypotension
  - *Nitrates*—Used to dilate coronary arteries and decrease/eliminate chest pain—can cause hypotension, tachycardias
  - *Glaucoma medications*—Used to decrease intraocular pressure—can cause bradycardias
  - *Erectile dysfunction medications*—Used to enable males to obtain/maintain an erection—can cause profound decrease in blood pressure, which can cause chest pain, myocardial ischemia, or MI
  - *Thrombolytics*—Used to abort a STEMI in progress—dissolves the blood clot causing the MI—can cause tachycardias if bleeding results—should cause elevated ST segment to return to normal
  - *Anticoagulants*—Blood thinners—used to prevent blood clots—can cause tachycardias if bleeding results
- **Pacemakers**—Used to speed up (or in some cases slow down) the heart rate
- **Permanent pacemakers are implanted into the body.**
- **Temporary pacemakers can be temporarily inserted into or externally attached to the body.**

- **Pacemaker terminology:**
  - *Firing*—Pacemaker's generation of an impulse—results in pacemaker spike on EKG
  - *Capture*—Chamber responds to pacemaker signal by depolarizing—results in P wave and /or QRS following pacer spike
  - *Sensing*—Pacemaker's ability to sense patient's underlying rhythm to determine if it needs to fire—results in appropriate delay before next paced beat on EKG
- **Pacemaker code:**
  - *First letter*—Chamber paced
  - *Second letter*—Chamber sensed
  - *Third letter*—Response to sensed events
- **VVI pacemaker**—Paces and senses the ventricle
- **DDD pacemaker**—Paces and senses atrium and ventricle
- **Pacemaker malfunctions:**
  - *Failure to fire*—No pacer spikes noted
  - *Loss of capture*—Spikes present, but no P or QRS following them
  - *Undersensing*—Pacer spikes inside QRS complexes or T waves
- **Cardiac Resynchronization Therapy**—utilizes a biventricular pacemaker to provide ventricular synchrony—used for symptomatic CHF patients with EF <35%, sinus rhythm with LBBB with QRS >0.13 secs wide—improves quality of life, increases EF by 10%, narrows the QRS complex, decreases left ventricular size
- **Electrical cardioversion**—Electrical shock using synchronizer button—shock is synchronized with cardiac cycle
- **Defibrillation**—Electric shock delivered immediately upon pressing button—normal treatment for V-fib and pulseless V-tach; not synchronized
- **Monitor-defibrillator**—Used in hospitals—can monitor different leads and can cardiovert/defib patient
- **AICD**—Implanted defibrillator—programmed to shock certain arrhythmias
- **AED**—Defibrillator found in public areas such as airports—for use by lay public
- **Therapeutic hypothermia**—Cooling the post–cardiac arrest patient down to 90 to 93 degrees Fahrenheit—helps improve neurologic function and provides better outcomes. During cool-down period: atrial and ventricular arrhythmias common. Sinus tach common at first, slowing to sinus brady as temperature drops further. During warm-up phase: watch for hyperkalemia—tall pointy T waves and widening QRS complexes.

Practice Quiz

1. Digitalis is classified as which kind of medication? _____

2. Class I antiarrhythmic medications have which effect on the action potential? _____

3. What effect does atropine have on the heart rate? _____

4. What effect does vasoconstriction have on the blood pressure? _____

5. True or false: An AED is meant for use by lay people.

6. What effect do class III antiarrhythmic medications have on the action potential? _____

7. Explain the use of therapeutic hypothermia. _____

8. Explain what the three letters of the pacemaker code refer to. _____

9. How does cardioversion differ from defibrillation? _____

10. Describe antitachycardia pacing and how it differs from routine pacing for bradycardias. _____

Putting It All Together—Critical Thinking Exercises

These exercises may consist of diagrams to label, scenarios to analyze, brain-stumping questions to ponder, or other exercises to help boost your understanding of the chapter material.

1. For the following "shockable" rhythms, state whether the rhythm should be cardioverted or defibrillated:

   a. Atrial fibrillation _____

   b. Ventricular tachycardia with a pulse _____

   c. Ventricular fibrillation _____

   d. Ventricular tachycardia without a pulse _____

   e. SVT _____

2. The following scenario will provide you with information about a fictional patient and ask you to analyze the situation, answer questions, and decide on appropriate actions.

   Mr. Johnson had a temporary transvenous VVI pacemaker inserted yesterday because of slow atrial fibrillation. It's set at a rate of 60. This morning he calls you to his room complaining of feeling faint. His blood pressure has dropped and his rhythm is as seen on the strip that follows. See Figure 4–14.

   a. What is this rhythm and heart rate? _____

   b. What is the pacemaker doing? _____

   c. Describe how to utilize the pacemaker to abolish this rhythm. _____

   _____

   _____

   _____

   Within a few minutes, Mr. Johnson's rhythm has changed. See Figure 4–15. His blood pressure remains low and he still feels faint.

   d. What is this rhythm and heart rate? _____

   e. What is the pacemaker doing? _____

   f. Is there a pacer malfunction? Explain. _____

   _____

   _____

   g. What corrective measures can help remedy the pacer malfunction? _____

   _____

   _____

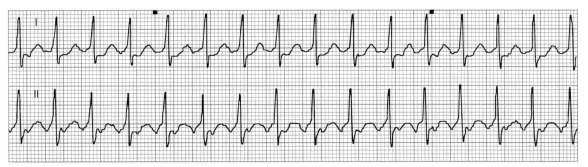

FIGURE 4–14

Mr. Johnson's first rhythm strip.

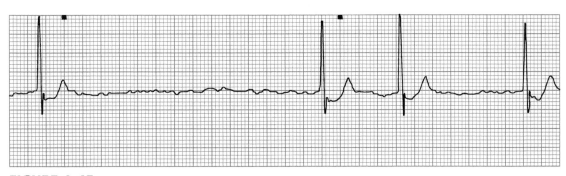

FIGURE 4–15

Mr. Johnson's second strip.

h. Explain the physiological reason that he had low blood pressure and a feeling of faintness with both rhythms seen on his rhythm strips.

_____

_____

After corrective measures, the pacemaker now works properly, and Mr. Johnson is in paced rhythm with a good blood pressure. He feels much better.

3. How did you do with these questions? Let's do one more scenario.

Mr. Lohtrip is a 65-year-old male with a history of diabetes and erectile dysfunction. His medications are sildenafil and insulin. Tonight, as usual, he experienced mild chest pressure after sexual intercourse with his wife, but this time it didn't go away spontaneously as it usually did, so he took one of his wife's nitroglycerin tablets. Shortly after taking the nitro, Mr. Lohtrip collapsed. His wife called 911 and the ambulance took him to the hospital where his heart rate is noted to be 135, BP low at 68/30, and his 12-lead EKG shows he is having an MI.

a. What do you suspect is causing his tachycardia, low BP, and MI? _____

_____

_____

b. What would you teach Mr. Lohtrip in the future about his medications? _____

_____

_____

Putting It All Together: Critical Thinking Scenarios

CHAPTER 5 OBJECTIVES

Upon completion of this chapter, the student will be able to

- Correlate certain rhythms and 12-lead EKGs with their treatment.
- Demonstrate critical thinking skills.

What It's All About

Mr. Coleman was in the midst of an inferior MI, as evidenced by ST segment elevation in Leads II, III, and aVF on the 12-lead EKG he'd just had done. He was having typical symptoms of an MI—chest heaviness, shortness of breath, nausea, and diaphoresis. But Mr. Coleman's blood pressure was also very low—not typical of an uncomplicated inferior MI. The ED tech did a right-sided EKG and confirmed that Mr. Coleman's inferior wall MI had extended into his right ventricle. The cardiologist and the cardiac cath lab team were notified to come to the hospital and Mr. Coleman was taken to the cardiac cath lab where he underwent a PCI procedure. He recovered uneventfully.

Introduction

Throughout the previous chapters, you've been working with practice skills and critical thinking exercises to boost your understanding of the chapter material. In the following scenarios, you will use every skill you have. You will analyze rhythms and 12-lead EKGs and decide on a course of action. What's going on? Why is it happening? What was done about it in the scenario? What *should have* been done? Is there an MI? What's the rhythm? What medication and/or electrical therapy is indicated? This is the pinnacle of the learning experience—not just mindlessly memorizing material, but using it in a practical way. Let's get started.

Scenario A: Mr. Johnson

Mr. Johnson, age 52, was admitted to the hospital's telemetry floor complaining of mild chest discomfort that had lasted 2 hours and was unrelieved by antacids. Both of his parents had a history of heart disease, so Mr. Johnson was afraid he might be having a heart attack. His initial EKG in the emergency department was completely normal, and his pain was relieved with one sublingual nitroglycerin tablet. Medical history included a two-pack-a-day cigarette habit, as well as major surgery the previous week to remove a small colon cancer. Mr. Johnson had been asleep in his room for about an hour when the nurse observed the strip shown in Figure 5–1 on his cardiac monitor.

1. What do you see of concern on the rhythm strip in Figure 5–1? _____

_____

The nurse went to check on Mr. Johnson and found him just awakening and complaining of a dull ache in his chest. Per unit protocol, the nurse did a 12-lead EKG, shown in Figure 5–2.

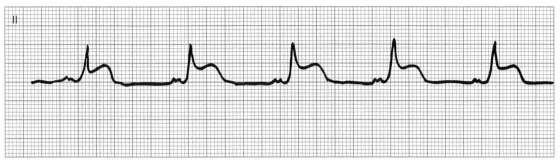

FIGURE 5–1

Mr. Johnson's rhythm.

2. What conclusion do you draw from the EKG in Figure 5–2? _____
   _____

3. Mr. Johnson was moved to the coronary care unit and was started on a nitroglycerin
   infusion. For what purpose was this infusion started? _____
   _____

4. Mr. Johnson was also started on oxygen by nasal prongs. What beneficial effect
   would the oxygen be expected to have? _____

5. The physician considered starting thrombolytic therapy (their small community
   hospital didn't have a cardiac cath lab to do PCI), but because of Mr. Johnson's
   recent surgery decided he was not a candidate for thrombolytics. What is the mode
   of action of thrombolytic medications? _____
   _____

6. What is the danger of giving thrombolytics to someone who had recent
   surgery? _____
   _____

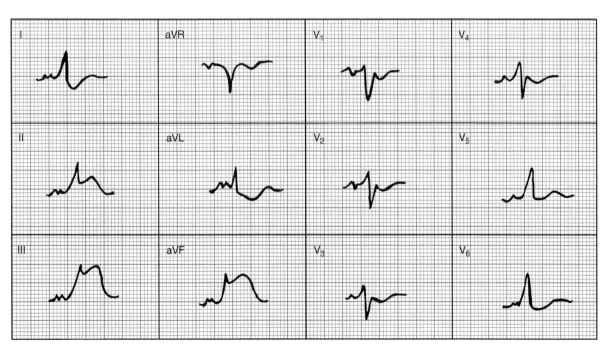

FIGURE 5–2

Mr. Johnson's 12-lead EKG done during chest pain.

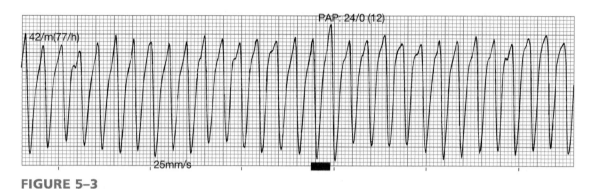

FIGURE 5–3

Mr. Johnson's second rhythm strip.

Shortly after arrival in the CCU, Mr. Johnson called his nurse and told her he felt "funny." He denied pain but stated he felt "full in the head." The nurse noticed the rhythm in Figure 5–3 on the monitor in Mr. Johnson's room.

7. What is the rhythm shown in Figure 5–3? _____

8. Mr. Johnson's arrhythmia spontaneously converted back to sinus rhythm without treatment. The nurse notified the physician, who ordered labs to be drawn. What electrolyte abnormality can cause this rhythm? _____

9. What other blood abnormality can cause this rhythm? _____

10. What medications could have been used to treat this arrhythmia if it had continued? _____

Mr. Johnson's lab work revealed a very low potassium level. He was given supplemental potassium intravenously, and his arrhythmia did not recur. His blood oxygen level was normal.

Shortly after breakfast the next morning, Mr. Johnson developed midsternal chest pain (pain under the center of the breastbone) radiating to his left arm. The pain was severe, and he became diaphoretic and complained of mild nausea. His nurse gave him a sublingual nitroglycerin tablet and increased the rate of his nitroglycerin infusion.

11. What is another medication that could be given to treat Mr. Johnson's chest pain? _____

_____

12. A 12-lead EKG was done stat (immediately) and is seen in Figure 5–4. What conclusion do you draw from this EKG? _____

Within 15 minutes, Mr. Johnson's pain was gone but his blood pressure was low and his rhythm had changed. See Figure 5–5 for his next rhythm.

13. What is the rhythm in Figure 5–5? _____

14. What effect does this rhythm have on cardiac output? _____

15. What is the appropriate treatment for this rhythm? _____

16. Where are the possible sites of the block? _____

17. If the block were at the bundle branches, what effect would atropine have? _____

_____

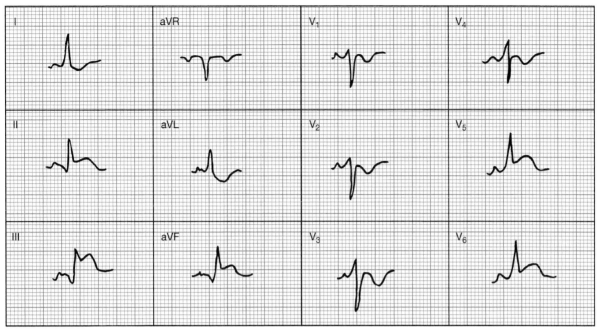

FIGURE 5–4

Mr. Johnson's second 12-lead EKG.

After the appropriate treatment was given, Mr. Johnson's blood pressure returned to normal, and his rhythm was as seen in Figure 5–6.

18. What rhythm is shown in Figure 5–6? _____

19. What symptoms, if any, would you expect Mr. Johnson to have with this rhythm? _____

_____

Concerned about the implications of the most recent EKG and his arrhythmias, Mr. Johnson's physician conferred with cardiologists at a large teaching hospital 60 miles away. Soon Mr. Johnson was transferred by helicopter to that hospital and taken straight to its cardiac catheterization lab, where an emergency angiogram was done. It revealed significant blockage in two of his coronary arteries.

20. Based on the two EKGs in Figures 5–2 and 5–4, which two coronary arteries do you suspect might be blocked? _____

PCI was attempted but was unsuccessful, so Mr. Johnson was taken to the operating room to have bypass surgery. He recovered uneventfully.

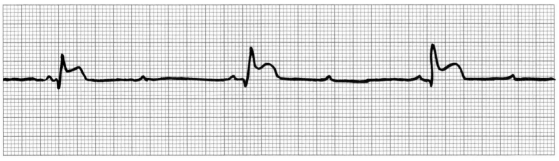

FIGURE 5–5

Mr. Johnson's third rhythm strip.

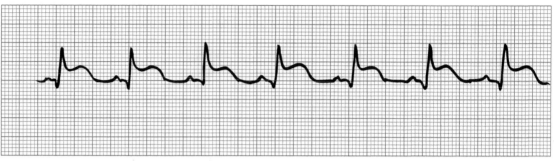

FIGURE 5–6

Mr. Johnson's fourth rhythm strip.

Scenario B: Ms. Capitano

Ms. Capitano was a 23-year-old woman who presented to the ER with complaints of fatigue and dizziness. She had a negative medical history and did not smoke. Aside from birth control pills, she took no medication and denied illegal drug use. She did drink five or six soft drinks daily and had two to three cups of coffee every morning. Cardiac monitor revealed the rhythm seen in Figure 5–7.

1. What is the rhythm shown in Figure 5–7? _____

2. What is the likely cause of this rhythm in Ms. Capitano's case? _____
   _____

3. The physician ordered adenosine to be given intravenously. The rhythm strip shown in Figure 5–8 was the result. What happened? _____
   _____

After a few seconds of the slow heart rate, Ms. Capitano's heart rate sped back up—to the 250s this time—and she complained of feeling faint. Her blood pressure, which had been normal at 110/60, plummeted to 68/50, and she was now pale and drenched in sweat.

4. What effect was the tachycardia having on her cardiac output? _____
   _____

Ms. Capitano's condition had worsened—she was now in shock. The ER physician elected to perform synchronized electrical cardioversion. After a low-voltage shock, Ms. Capitano's rhythm converted to sinus rhythm with a heart rate in the 90s and her blood pressure improved. Soon her color was back to normal and her skin was dry. She was admitted to the coronary care unit for close observation and was started on calcium channel blockers to prevent recurrences of her tachycardia. The physician advised her to curtail her caffeine intake. After a day in CCU, Ms. Capitano was transferred to the telemetry floor. She was sent home a day later, doing well.

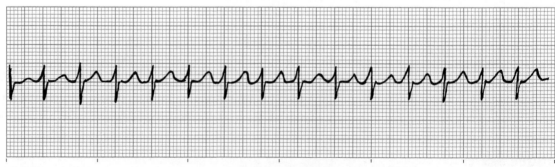

FIGURE 5–7

Ms. Capitano's initial rhythm in the ER.

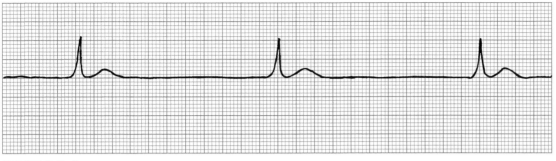

FIGURE 5–8

Ms. Capitano's rhythm after adenosine administration.

Scenario C: Mr. Farley

A few years ago, Mr. Farley had been diagnosed with atrial fibrillation and was started on digitalis. He'd done well, with a heart rate running in the 70s and 80s since then. For the past few days, however, Mr. Farley had felt lousy—nothing specific, just "not right," as he would later describe it. He didn't think it was important enough to bother his physician, although his wife had fussed at him to do so. Believing his problem to be related to his atrial fibrillation, Mr. Farley doubled up on his digitalis dose. If one pill a day was good, two a day had to be better, he reasoned. After five days of this, he began suffering from violent nausea and vomiting episodes. His wife dragged the reluctant Mr. Farley to the hospital. His initial rhythm strip is shown in Figure 5–9.

1. What is the rhythm in Figure 5–9? _____

2. What effect does this rhythm have on the atrial kick? _____

   _____

3. Lab tests revealed that the level of digitalis in Mr. Farley's bloodstream was at toxic levels. Name three rhythms that can be caused by digitalis toxicity. _____

   _____

The physician contemplated sending Mr. Farley to the CCU, but because his blood pressure was good and he looked OK, he was sent to the telemetry floor instead. His nausea was treated with medication and he was taken off digitalis. Three hours after arriving on the telemetry floor, Mr. Farley passed out in the bathroom. His new rhythm is shown in Figure 5–10.

4. What is the rhythm in Figure 5–10? _____

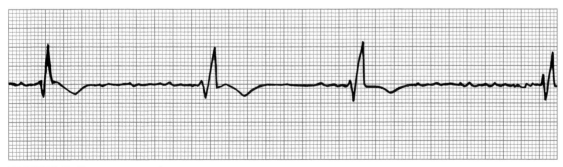

FIGURE 5–9

Mr. Farley's initial rhythm strip.

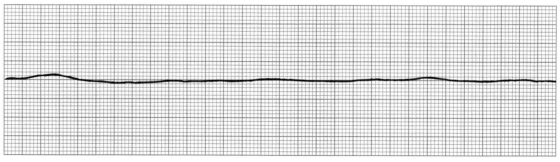

FIGURE 5–10

Mr. Farley's second rhythm strip.

5. The emergency team was called and CPR was initiated. What medication would be appropriate to give at this time? _____

_____

6. After successful resuscitation, Mr. Farley was transferred to the CCU, where a temporary transvenous pacemaker was inserted. What beneficial effect would the pacemaker have? _____

_____

7. A few hours after the pacemaker was inserted, the nurse noticed evidence of loss of capture on the monitor. On the monitor strip in Figure 5–11, what would tell her there was loss of capture? _____

_____

8. What can be done to restore capture? _____

_____

   Capture was restored, and Mr. Farley rested well for the next few hours. Suddenly, he went into V-tach with a heart rate of 200. The nurses could tell by the deflection of the QRS complexes that the V-tach was originating in the left ventricle, so they knew it was not induced by irritation from the pacemaker wire in the right ventricle.

9. With a pacemaker in place, what can be done to terminate the tachycardia? _____

_____

10. With the V-tach now resolved, Mr. Farley was started on an amiodarone infusion to prevent a recurrence of the V-tach. What is amiodarone's effect on the ventricle? _____

_____

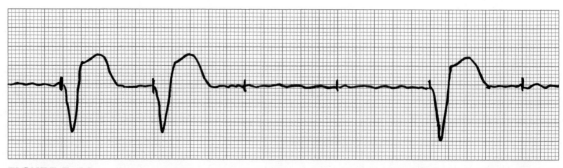

FIGURE 5–11

Mr. Farley's third rhythm strip.

11. The rest of Mr. Farley's hospital stay was uneventful. Because his problem began with his inappropriate self-dosing of digitalis, what would you tell Mr. Farley regarding his digitalis dose in the future? _____

Scenario D: Mr. Lew

Mr. Lew, age 78, had never been in the hospital and had not seen his physician in 7 years. By all accounts, he was unusually healthy for his age. He was not alarmed by the occasional tightness in his chest—and in fact took it as a sign that he was out of shape and needed to exercise more. One summer day, while he was mowing the lawn, his chest tightness came back, but this time it was much more intense, and Mr. Lew became concerned. He called his son to take him to the hospital. On the way, Mr. Lew passed out in the car and slumped over onto his son, causing an accident. Ambulances rushed the duo to the closest ER. Stephen, the son, was treated for a fractured arm and was discharged in a cast. Although not injured in the accident, Mr. Lew was in much worse shape. See his EKG in Figure 5–12.

1. What conclusion do you draw from the EKG in Figure 5–12? _____

_____

Mr. Lew's condition was precarious. His blood pressure was low and he was in danger of cardiac arrest. Thrombolytic therapy was started (PCI was not possible at this small local hospital) and within one hour Mr. Lew's blood pressure had improved. Soon he was in the rhythm shown in Figure 5–13.

2. What is the rhythm in Figure 5–13? _____

_____

3. What, if any, treatment does this rhythm require in this case? _____

4. What in the past was thought to be the significance of this rhythm? _____

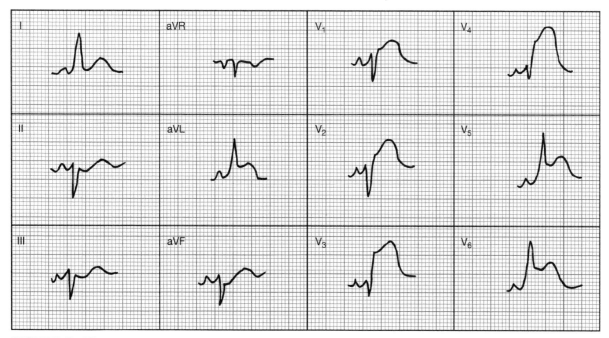

FIGURE 5–12

Mr. Lew's initial 12-lead EKG.

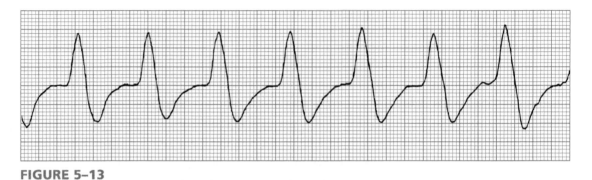

FIGURE 5–13

Mr. Lew's rhythm strip after thrombolytic therapy.

This rhythm converted back to sinus rhythm within 30 minutes. Mr. Lew's condition improved over the next hour, and he was transferred to the coronary care unit, where he stabilized.

When Stephen came by to see his dad the next day, Mr. Lew whispered to him that he was having mild chest pain again, but that it wasn't bad enough to bother the nurses. Stephen alerted the nurse, who did an EKG while the pain was in progress. See the EKG in Figure 5–14.

5. What conclusion do you draw from the EKG in Figure 5–14? _____

_____

Mr. Lew's nitroglycerin infusion was adjusted and he was taken for an emergency angiogram. An occlusion of the left main coronary artery was noted, along with blockage in another coronary artery.

6. Based on the two EKGs in Figures 5–12 and 5–14, which other coronary artery is involved? _____

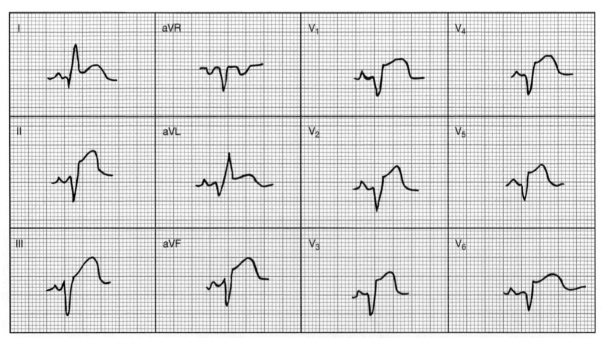

FIGURE 5–14

Mr. Lew's EKG done during chest pain.

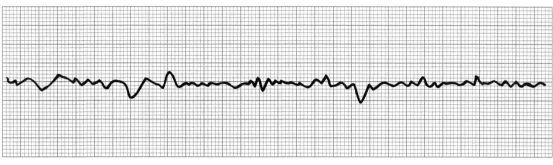

FIGURE 5–15

Mr. Lew's rhythm during cardiac arrest.

7. What is the cause of the ST segment depression noted on Mr. Lew's first EKG? _____

_____

Mr. Lew was taken to the operating room for emergency bypass surgery. Following cardiac arrest in the operating room, he returned to the CCU in critical condition. Within minutes Mr. Lew was in cardiac arrest again. The cardiac surgeon opened the chest sutures and did manual chest compressions by squeezing Mr. Lew's heart in his hands. Mr. Lew's rhythm strip is shown in Figure 5–15.

8. What is the rhythm in Figure 5–15? _____

Internal defibrillator paddles were inserted into the open chest cavity and placed on either side of Mr. Lew's heart. A small volt was discharged, and Mr. Lew's rhythm changed to the one shown in Figure 5–16.

9. What is the rhythm in Figure 5–16? _____

CPR was started again, and the staff administered various medications as well as temporary pacing, but Mr. Lew succumbed to his illness.

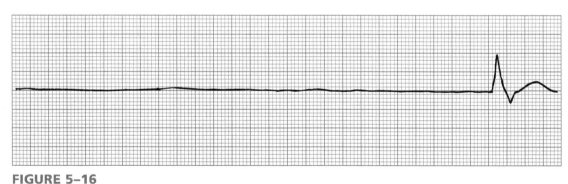

FIGURE 5–16

Mr. Lew's rhythm after defibrillation.

Scenario E: Mrs. Epstein

Mrs. Epstein had her pacemaker implanted 4 years ago because of third-degree AV block. She'd been doing well until this morning, when she began to feel dizzy. She took her pulse as she'd been taught to do and found it to be 38. Her rate-responsive DDD

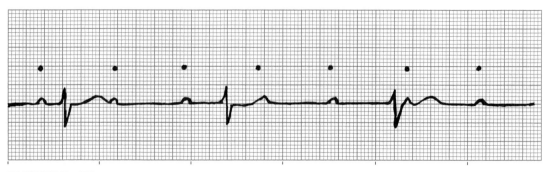

FIGURE 5–17

Mrs. Epstein's rhythm during a dizzy spell in the hospital.

pacemaker was set at a rate of 60 to 125. At the physician's office, the cardiologist found that the pacemaker needed a new battery. Because her heart rate was now in the 60s, he thought the battery change could wait until the next morning. He sent Mrs. Epstein to the hospital, where she was admitted to the telemetry floor.

A few hours after arrival, Mrs. Epstein complained again of dizziness, this time much worse. Her rhythm is shown in Figure 5–17.

1. What is the rhythm in Figure 5–17? _____

2. What is her pacemaker doing? _____

3. What is the likely cause of this problem? _____

The nurse, following hospital protocol, gave atropine and called for her coworkers to bring in the transcutaneous pacemaker. The pacemaker was attached and set on demand mode at a rate of 60.

After notifying the cardiologist of the situation, the nurse rushed Mrs. Epstein to the cardiac catheterization lab, where an emergency pacemaker battery change was done. After her return to the telemetry floor, the nurse noted her rhythm as shown in Figure 5–18.

4. What is the rhythm in Figure 5–18? _____

5. Is the pacemaker functioning properly? If not, what is the problem? _____
_____

Mrs. Epstein was discharged the following day in good condition.

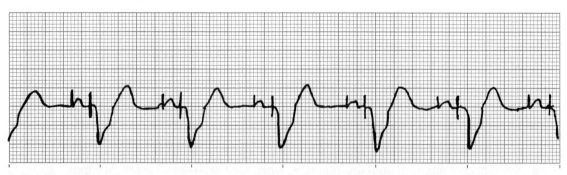

FIGURE 5–18

Mrs. Epstein's rhythm on return from her pacemaker battery change.

Scenario F: Mr. Calico

Mr. Calico, age 76, was taking a walk when he developed chest heaviness. He went inside and told his wife he was going to lie down on the sofa for a while. She grew concerned an hour later when she called his name and he didn't answer. Mrs. Calico called 911 and the paramedics arrived to find Mr. Calico in the rhythm seen in Figure 5–19.

1. What is this rhythm? _____

2. What symptoms would you expect to see in Mr. Calico? _____

3. Mr. Calico was unconscious and had no pulse and no breathing. What should the paramedics do to resuscitate Mr. Calico? _____

   After appropriate initial treatment, Mr. Calico's pulse returned and he began to awaken. The paramedics ran another rhythm strip. See Figure 5–20.

4. What is this rhythm? _____

   Paramedics rushed Mr. Calico to the nearest hospital, where a 12-lead EKG was done. His 12-lead EKG is seen in Figure 5–21.

5. What conclusion do you draw from this EKG? _____

6. Thrombolytic medication was started and the EKG was repeated. See Figure 5–22. What has changed since the last EKG? _____

7. Mr. Calico went into ventricular fibrillation a few minutes later. The nurse prepared to cardiovert the rhythm, but when he depressed the buttons to deliver the shock, nothing happened. Why and what corrective action is needed for this problem?

   _____

   After correctly defibrillating Mr. Calico, the ER staff sent him to the CCU, where he spent a week recovering. He went home and did well with no further problems.

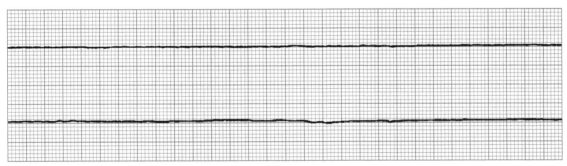

FIGURE 5–19

Mr. Calico's initial rhythm.

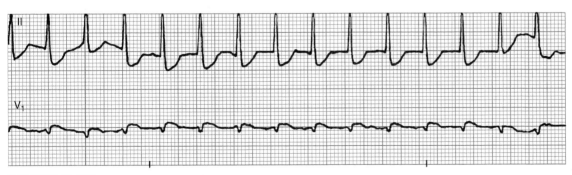

FIGURE 5–20

Mr. Calico's rhythm after initial treatment.

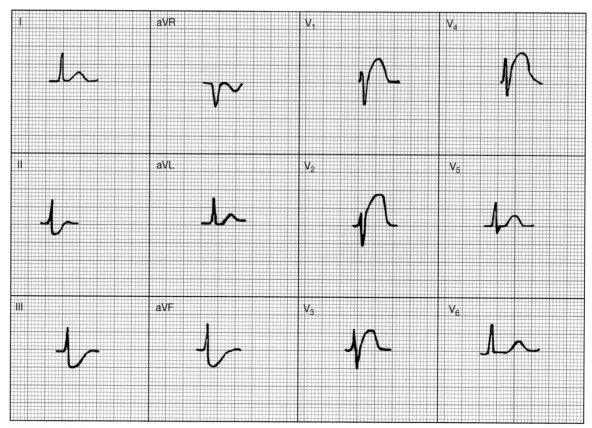

FIGURE 5–21

Mr. Calico's initial 12-lead EKG.

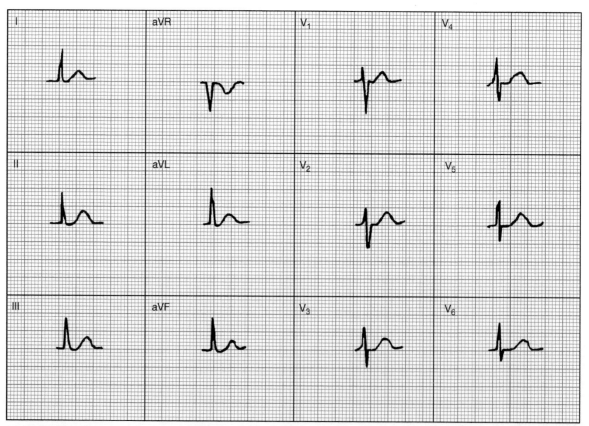

FIGURE 5–22

Mr. Calico's EKG after thrombolytic medication.

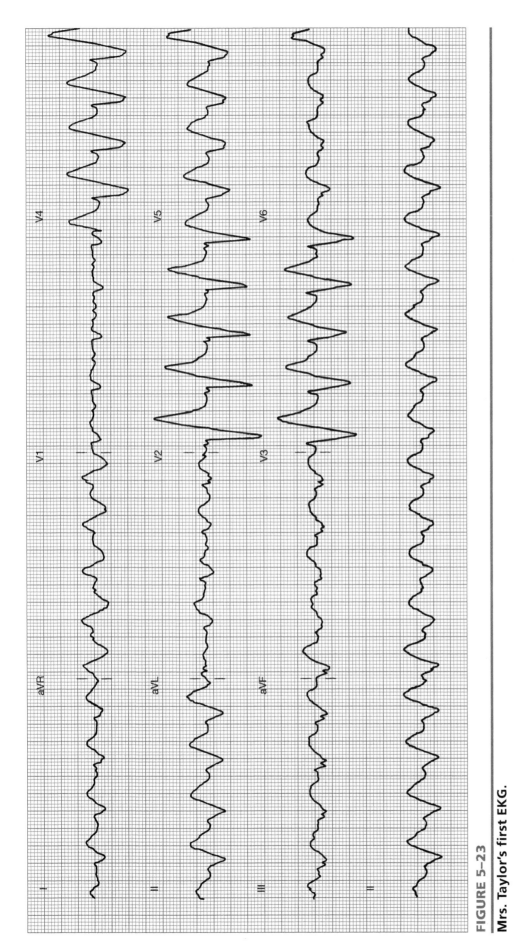

FIGURE 5–23

Mrs. Taylor's first EKG.

Scenario G: Mrs. Taylor

Mrs. Taylor, age 45, had been in kidney failure for 15 years and had required dialysis for most of that time. Because of other health problems (diabetes, heart disease, asthma), she was told she was not a candidate for a kidney transplant. At her local hospital, Mrs. Taylor was notorious for coming in critically ill after skipping two or three dialysis treatments. She'd be admitted to the intensive care unit, treated, and released a week or so later, with a warning not to skip dialysis any more. But a few months later she'd be back again.

Tonight Mrs. Taylor comes in yet again. Her potassium level is 8.9, dangerously high. Her EKG is shown in Figure 5–23.

1. Elevated potassium levels can cause two main effects on the EKG. What are they and which one or ones do you see on this EKG? _____
   _____

Almost immediately after arrival in the ER, Mrs. Taylor loses consciousness and suffers cardiac arrest. The nurse records the following rhythm strip as she begins CPR. See Figure 5–24.

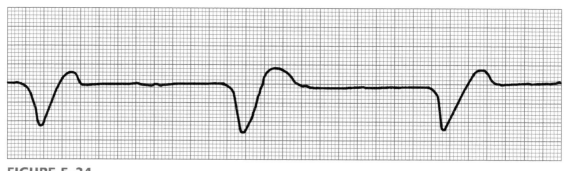

FIGURE 5–24

Mrs. Taylor's rhythm strip during cardiac arrest.

2. What is this rhythm? _____

The physician orders calcium to be given intravenously. Calcium decreases the potassium level in the bloodstream. After giving the calcium, the nurse runs the following EKG. See Figure 5–25.

3. What change do you see in the QRS complex? _____

Mrs. Taylor's pulse and breathing resume after the calcium. She is sent to the intensive care unit, where she undergoes dialysis. Four days later, she is well enough to go home. Once again she is warned that the next time she skips dialysis, it could be fatal. She smiles at the nurses and says, "I know, I know."

Scenario H: Mr. Foster

Mr. Foster was a 28-year-old male who'd been abusing cocaine for years. Tonight he and some friends had been "partying" with various substances—cocaine, ecstasy, and other drugs—when Mr. Foster began to complain of chest pain. His friends were alarmed when Mr. Foster clutched his chest and curled into a ball on the ground, moaning in pain. They pulled him up and brought him to the hospital. A 12-lead EKG was done and is shown in Figure 5–26.

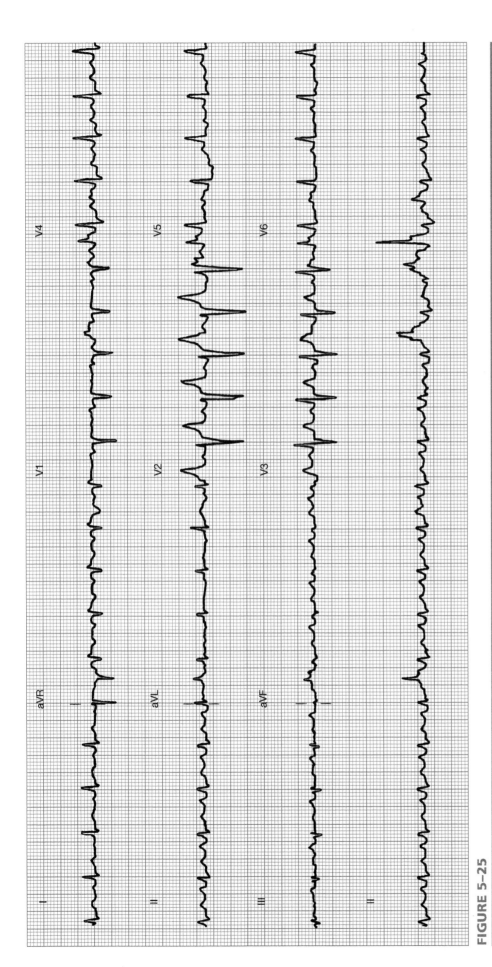

FIGURE 5–25

Mrs. Taylor's EKG after calcium.

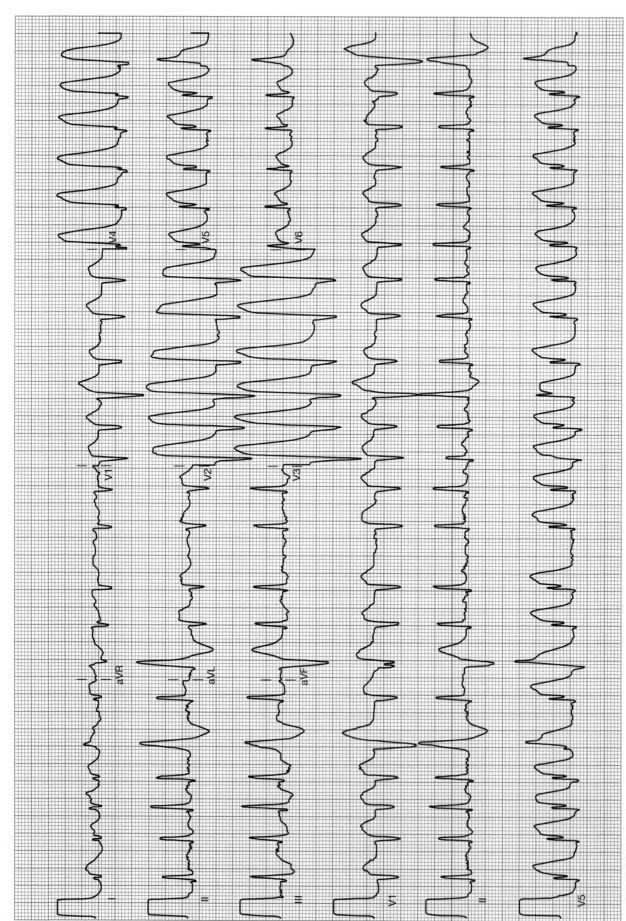

FIGURE 5–26

Mr. Foster's 12-lead EKG.

1. What is Mr. Foster's rhythm and heart rate? _____

Mr. Foster is initially unable to answer questions about his medical condition or history and the staff are unable to contact family. The ER nurse asks the physician if she wants to do elective cardioversion to convert the rhythm to sinus. The physician says no.

2. Why would she not want to shock this rhythm at this time? _____

3. There is evidence of an MI on the EKG. Is it a STEMI or a non-STEMI? _____

4. Which wall or walls of the heart is/are infarcted? _____
_____

Mr. Foster is started on oxygen and given an aspirin tablet to chew. He is then given a nitroglycerin pill sublingually and the pain starts to decrease, as does his heart rate—it drops to a mean rate in the 80s. The physician advises Mr. Foster that he is having an MI and Mr. Foster is incredulous. "But I'm only 28, man! Heart attacks are for old people!" The physician explains that cocaine use greatly increases the chance of an MI even in young people who would not otherwise be considered high risk. The cardiac cath lab team is called out and Mr. Foster is taken for an angiogram, which is completely normal.

5. What effect of cocaine can cause an MI in patients with no coronary artery disease?
_____

Mr. Foster is sent to the ICU and recovers uneventfully. He is discharged and immediately goes into rehab to address his drug habit. The cardiologist tells him "this cocaine-induced coronary artery spasm gave you a heart attack at age 28. The next one could kill you."

Scenario I: Mr. Frye

Mr. Frye was at work one evening when he developed shortness of breath and palpitations—"it felt like a fish flopping around in my chest," he described it later. Mr. Frye drove himself to the ER, where he was attached to a cardiac monitor, started on oxygen, and had an IV inserted. The physician evaluated Mr. Frye's heart rhythm.
See Figure 5–27.

1. What is this rhythm? _____

2. What's the heart rate? _____

Vagal maneuvers were suggested as a method of terminating the rhythm.

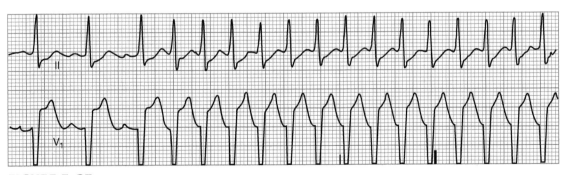

FIGURE 5–27

Mr. Frye's rhythm.

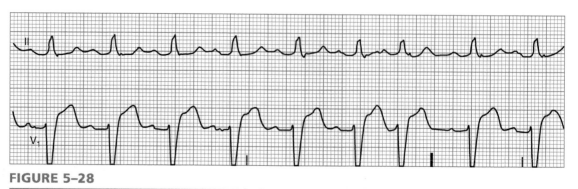

FIGURE 5–28

Mr. Frye's rhythm following the second dose of adenosine.

3. What effect does stimulation of the vagus nerve have on the heart rate? _____

Vagal maneuvers were unsuccessful. His heart rate was still tachycardic and he was looking more and more pale. His blood pressure was 100/50—a bit below his normal of 110/70. The ER physician ordered adenosine to be given IV. Everyone watched the heart monitor as the adenosine was injected into the IV line. No change. A second dose of adenosine—double the first dose—was given. See Figure 5–28 for Mr. Frye's rhythm following the second dose of adenosine.

4. What do you see on this strip? _____

5. What unnerving side effect can adenosine have on the rhythm and heart rate? _____
    _____

6. Was that effect evident in Figure 5–28? _____

After the second dose of the medication, Mr. Frye's skin dried up, his color returned, and his shortness of breath was gone.

7. What other treatments would have been appropriate for Mr. Frye's initial rhythm? ___
    _____

Scenario J: Mrs. Terry

Mr. and Mrs. Terry were at the mall when Mrs. Terry, age 38, felt a crushing fatigue. Let's just go home—I want to lie down, she told her husband. Later Mrs. Terry became woozy and very pale. Her husband, concerned his wife might have the flu, took her to the hospital. The nurse inquired about any medications she was on and whether or not she was a smoker. Mrs. Terry answered that her only med was a daily birth control pill and she acknowledged that she smoked two packs of cigarettes per day. The ER physician examined her and agreed with Mr. Terry. "I think you probably just picked up the flu bug," he told her. "There's not much to do but ride it out. Just stay in bed a few days and you should feel better." So they went home and Mrs. Terry climbed into bed. The next morning she felt worse—short of breath now—so she called her family doctor and went to his office. He examined her and told her he also thought she had the flu. "You'll probably feel worse before you feel better," he told her. "Just go to bed and wait it out." So off they went back home. Mrs. Terry went straight to bed while her hubby watched TV. Mr. Terry checked in on his wife a few hours later and found her barely conscious. He called 911 and the paramedics arrived and attached Mrs. Terry to the cardiac monitor, which revealed the following rhythm. See Figure 5–29.

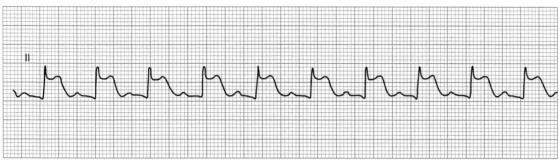

FIGURE 5–29

Mrs. Terry's rhythm strip.

1. What is the rhythm and heart rate? _____

2. Are there any other abnormalities on this strip? If so, what? _____
   _____

   The paramedics rushed Mrs. Terry to the closest ER. Enroute, they did a 12-lead EKG and transmitted it to the hospital. See Figure 5–30.

3. What abnormalities does this EKG show? _____

4. Assuming the hospital is suitably equipped to handle this, what is the preferred treatment for this condition, according to the American College of Cardiology and the American Heart Association? _____

5. Mrs. Terry was found to have a large occlusion in a coronary artery. Based on the EKG, which coronary artery do you suspect was involved? _____

   She was successfully treated. After assessing her risk factors for heart disease, the cardiologist concluded that Mrs. Terry's birth control pills, combined with her 2-pack-a-day smoking habit and her age, caused her MI. The cardiologist told her that her brand of birth control pills contains estrogen, known to increase the risk for blood clots, heart attacks, and strokes, especially in women over age 35 who smoke. And the vague symptoms were typical of females with MIs. The cardiologist told her that because of these vague symptoms and her age, there was no red flag to raise the doctors' suspicion of an MI—until she collapsed and was picked up by paramedics. That's why she'd been misdiagnosed twice with the flu.

   When she was sent home a week later, Mrs. Terry was advised to use an alternate form of birth control—no more birth control pills—and to avoid getting pregnant for at least a year in order to let her heart heal. Two years later, the Terrys became the proud parents of twin boys.

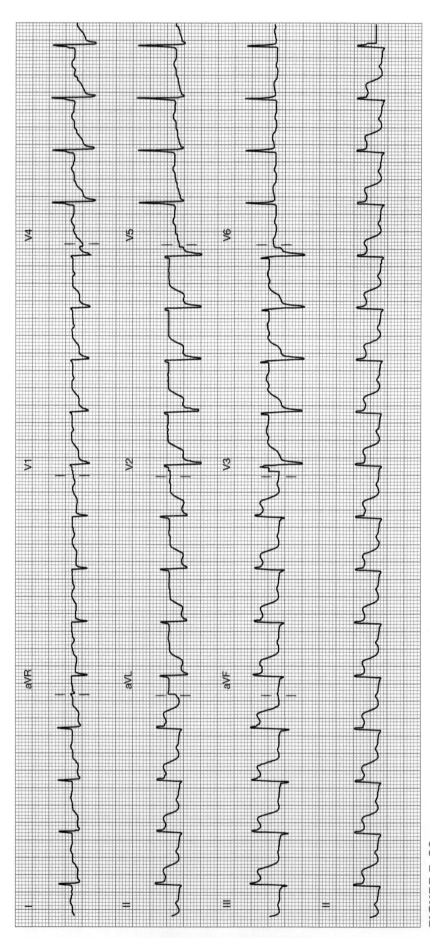

FIGURE 5–30

Mrs. Terry's EKG.

Appendix
Answers

CHAPTER ONE
Lead Morphology Practice

1. **Normal morphology.**
2. **Abnormal morphology.** Let's go lead by lead. Lead I is normal. Leads II and III are negative deflections, and they should be positive; aVR is OK, as is aVL; aVF is negative and it should be positive. The precordial leads are OK.
3. **Abnormal morphology.** Lead I is negative and it should be positive. Leads II and III are OK; aVR is positive and it should *always* be negative; aVL is negative and should be positive; aVF is OK. V_1 is positive but should be negative. V_2 is OK, more negative than positive. V_3 is positive but should be isoelectric. V_4 is isoelectric when it should be getting more positive. V_5 and V_6 are negative when they should be positive.
4. **Abnormal morphology.** Lead I is positive, as it should be. Leads II and III are negative but should be positive; aVR and aVL are OK; aVF is negative but should be positive. The precordial leads are all positive—this is completely abnormal.

Axis Practice EKGs

1. **Left axis deviation.** Lead I is positive and aVF is negative, so there is a left axis deviation.
2. **Normal axis.** Leads I and aVF are both positive, so the axis is in the normal quadrant.
3. **Indeterminate axis.** Leads I and aVF are both negative, so there is indeterminate axis.
4. **Left axis deviation.** Lead I is positive and aVF is negative, giving us a left axis deviation.
5. **Right axis deviation.** Lead I is negative and aVF is positive, so there is a right axis deviation.
6. **Normal axis.** Leads I and aVF are both positive, so the axis is in the normal quadrant.
7. **Normal axis.** Again, Leads I and aVF both are positive, so axis is normal.

BBB Practice

1. **No BBB. LAHB present**. The QRS interval is normal (about 0.10 seconds), so there is no BBB.

But there is a small Q in Lead I and a small R in Lead III, so there's a LAHB.
2. **RBBB and LAHB.** There is not the typical RSR' configuration in V_1—the initial R wave is missing—but it is still a RBBB. The QRS is wide (about 0.12 seconds) and the T wave slopes off opposite the final wave of the QRS complex. There is left axis deviation, which, in the presence of a RBBB, almost always implies a coexisting LAHB.
3. **LBBB**. There is a wide QRS (about 0.14 seconds), and a QS complex in V_1. The T wave is opposite the final part of the QRS.
4. **LBBB**. Again, there is a wide QRS of about 0.13 seconds, a QS in V_1. The T wave is opposite the final wave of the QRS complex.
5. **RBBB and LPHB**. There is a wide QRS with a QR configuration in V_1. Also there's a right axis deviation, which implies LPHB here.
6. **RBBB**. Note the RSR' configuration in V_1, along with the QRS interval of 0.12 seconds and the T wave opposite the terminal wave of the QRS. The axis here is indeterminate, which does not imply a hemiblock.
7. **LBBB**. Note the QS configuration in V_1 with the QRS interval of 0.14 seconds and the T wave opposite the terminal QRS wave.
8. **RBBB**. Note the RR' configuration in V_1 along with a QRS interval of about 0.12 seconds and a T wave opposite the terminal QRS wave. The indeterminate axis does not imply hemiblock.
9. **RBBB**. There's an RSR' in V_1, the QRS interval is 0.16 seconds, and the T wave is opposite the terminal QRS wave. Axis is normal, so no hemiblock.
10. **No BBB or HB**. The QRS interval is normal, about 0.08 seconds.

Hypertrophy Practice

1. **LVH.** The QRS in V_1 is about 8 mm deep, and the R wave in V_5 is 41 mm tall (it extends up beyond the QRS in V_4). Total is greater than

35 mm, so this EKG meets and exceeds the criteria for LVH.

2. **Low voltage.** The QRS complexes are short in all leads, especially aVL, which is tiny.

3. **Normal.** There is no hypertrophy or low voltage.

4. **RVH.** The R wave in V_1 is as tall as, if not slightly taller than, the S wave is deep and there is right axis deviation. The T wave is not inverted here as it often is, but that is not an absolute requirement for RVH.

5. **LVH.** The QRS in V_1 is 23 mm deep and in V_5 is 15 mm tall, for a total of 38 mm, more than enough to meet the voltage criteria for LVH.

Practice Quiz

1. If the QRS complexes in Leads I and aVF are both negative, **the axis is in the indeterminate axis quadrant.**

2. **False.** Right bundle branch block can be a normal variant, seen in normal hearts.

3. Sagging ST segments are associated with **digitalis effect.**

4. **False.** Tall pointy T waves are typical of hyper-kalemia, not RBBB.

5. Three causes of axis deviations are any three of the following: **normal variant, advanced pregnancy or obesity, myocardial infarction, hypertrophy, arhythmias, chronic lung disease,** and **pulmonary embolism.**

6. The voltage criteria for LVH is the following: **If the S wave in V_1 or V_2 (whichever is deeper) added to the R wave in V_5 or V_6 (whichever is taller) is greater than or equal to 35, there is LVH.**

7. **False.** RVH is not always associated with an inverted T wave.

8. Hypertrophy is **excessive growth of tissue.**

9. Hypokalemia **causes the T wave to flatten.**

10. In a BBB, the **QRS interval must be at least 0.12 seconds.**

Critical Thinking Exercises

1. If both bundle branches became blocked simultaneously and no lower pacemaker took over, the rhythm would initially be **P-wave asystole, then eventually asystole.** The sinus node, unaffected by the BBB, would continue sending out its impulses as usual for a while. This would provide the P waves. There would be no QRS complexes following these P waves because the bundle branch blocks would prevent the sinus

impulses from reaching the ventricles. Thus, the rhythm is initially P-wave asystole. Eventually the sinus node would slow down and stop, as it becomes more and more compromised by the lack of blood flow. Thus, the P waves would stop. This would be asystole. Remember, if there are no QRS complexes, there is no pulse and no blood flow. The sinus node, like all heart tissues, requires blood flow to function. Thus, the sinus node would eventually fail because of a lack of perfusion.

2.

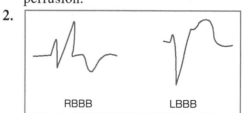

3. What happened is **she delivered the baby and her axis, which had been deviated to the left because of advanced pregnancy, is now back to normal.**

CHAPTER TWO
MI Practice

1. **Extensive anterior STEMI, acute**. Note the ST segment elevation in Leads I, aVL, and V_1 to V_6, along with reciprocal ST depression in II, III, and aVF. The T waves are upright.

2. **Inferior STEMI, age indeterminate**. Note the significant Q waves in II, III, and aVF, along with inverted T waves. The ST segment is at baseline. Remember, STEMIs develop Q waves as they evolve, and the ST segment retreats toward the baseline.

3. **Lateral wall STEMI, acute**. Note the ST elevation, significant Q waves, and inverted T waves in I, aVL, and V_5 to V_6, along with reciprocal ST depression in II, III, and aVF.

4. **Anteroseptal STEMI, acute**. Note the ST elevation and inverted T in V_1 to V_2, along with reciprocal ST depression in II, III, and aVF.

5. **No MI. Lateral wall ischemia present**. Note the T wave inversion in I, aVL, and V_5 to V_6. Remember that T wave inversion represents ischemia. There is no ST elevation or depression and no significant Q waves.

6. **Anteroseptal and inferior STEMI, both old**. Note the significant Q waves in V_1 to V_4 (anterior and septal leads), along with essentially normal ST segments. The ST does slope upward a bit in

V_1 to V_4, but it is not frankly elevated. There is also an old inferior MI. There are significant Q waves in III and aVF, but not in II; aVF is tiny, but you can see a Q wave there. That Q wave in aVF is significant because it is about half the size of the R wave—more than deep enough to meet the criteria. The T waves in the inferior leads are not inverted.

7. **Inferior and anterior-lateral STEMI, acute.** There is ST elevation in II, III, and aVF (inferior leads) and ST elevation and QS complexes in V_3 to V_6 (anterior and lateral leads). Leads V_1 and V_2 both have tiny R waves—those are not QS complexes there. It appears this patient started off with an anterior-lateral MI, which then extended into the inferior wall. The Q waves in V_3 to V_6 indicate that that infarct area is older than that in the inferior leads, where there are no significant Q waves.

8. **Inferior STEMI, acute.** There is ST elevation in II, III, and aVF, along with upright T waves and no significant Q waves as yet. Also note the reciprocal ST depression in I, aVL, and V_1 to V_3.

9. **Inferior-lateral STEMI, old.** There are significant Q waves in II, III, aVF (inferior leads), and V_6 (lateral lead) with upright T waves and baseline ST segments. Lead V_5 looks like it has a tiny R wave, not a Q wave. Also note the essentially nonexistent R wave progression in the precordial leads. This could imply an additional old anterior MI, or it could be caused by other factors.

10. **Inferior STEMI, acute.** Note the ST elevation in II, III, and aVF with reciprocal ST depression in I, aVL, and V_1 to V_3. There is a significant Q in III, but not yet in II or aVF.

Practice Quiz

1. The three I's of infarction are **ischemia, injury, and infarction.**
2. **A STEMI causes ST elevation, T wave inversion, and significant Q waves to develop on the EKG. The NSTEMI does not cause development of significant Q waves.**
3. Occlusion of the **left anterior descending coronary artery** causes anterior MI.
4. The normal indicative changes of an MI are **ST elevation, significant Q waves,** and **T wave inversions.**
5. Reciprocal changes are seen **in the area electrically opposite the damaged area.**
6. If there is ST elevation in II, III, and aVF, **the MI is acute inferior.**
7. If there is a significant Q wave in V_1 to V_3 with baseline ST segments and upright T waves, **the MI is an old anteroseptal MI.**
8. If the transition zone is in V_1 to V_2, **there is counterclockwise rotation of the heart.**
9. The kind of MI that can be diagnosed by inverting (turning over) the EKG and looking at Leads V_1 and V_2 from behind is the **posterior MI.**
10. The **circumflex coronary artery** supplies the lateral wall of the left ventricle.

Critical Thinking Exercises

1.
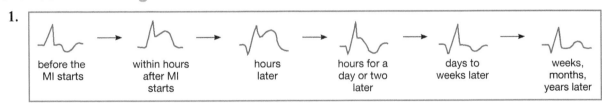

| before the MI starts | within hours after MI starts | hours later | hours for a day or two later | days to weeks later | weeks, months, years later |

2. If Mr. Milner, a 69-year-old man with a history of chest pain, arrives in your ER with newly inverted T waves in Leads II, III, and aVF, it is likely **he has new ischemia in the inferior wall of the left ventricle.**
3. If an hour later Mr. Milner is doubled over with crushing chest pain and his EKG now shows marked ST elevation in II, III, aVF, and V_{5-6}, **he is now injuring the inferior and lateral wall of the left ventricle.** This is an acute MI in progress, which is reversible if he receives PCI or thrombolytic medications. If the MI in progress is untreated, myocardial tissue will die and significant Q waves will develop in the inferior and lateral leads on his EKG.

4. Mr. Jones's EKG shows inverted T waves in II, III, and aVF—changes consistent with ischemia.

5. He is now having an MI. Leads II, III, and aVF show ST segment elevations and upright T waves. Notice that the T waves, which were inverted on the first EKG showing ischemia, now become upright. This is common once myocardial injury begins.

CHAPTER THREE
Practice EKGs

Note: For the intervals, it is acceptable if your answer is within 0.02 secs of displayed answer.

1.

- **Rhythm and rate:** Sinus rhythm with first-degree AV block, rate 62.
- **PR:** 0.20–0.24 **QRS:** 0.16 **QT:** 0.44–0.48.
- **Axis:** Normal. Both Leads I's and aVF's QRS complexes are positive.
- **BBB/HB:** Left bundle branch block.
- **Hypertrophy:** None.
- **Miscellaneous effects:** None. The widened QRS here is from the LBBB, not from hyperkalemia.
- **Infarction:** No evidence of ischemia or infarction.

2.

- **Rhythm and rate:** Sinus rhythm, rate 94.
- **PR:** 0.12 **QRS:** 0.06 **QT:** 0.34.
- **Axis:** Normal. I and aVF have positive QRSs.
- **BBB/HB:** None.
- **Hypertrophy:** None.
- **Miscellaneous effects:** None.
- **Infarction:** No evidence of ischemia or infarction.

3.

- **Rhythm and rate:** Sinus rhythm, rate 94.
- **PR:** 0.16 **QRS:** 0.14 **QT:** 0.40.
- **Axis:** Left axis deviation. Lead I is positive; aVF is negative.
- **BBB/HB:** RBBB and LAHB. A RBBB with a left axis deviation is almost always LAHB.
- **Hypertrophy:** None.
- **Miscellaneous effects:** None.
- **Infarction:** No evidence of ischemia or infarction. There is ST depression in many leads, but this is probably bundle related rather than true ischemia.

4.

- **Rhythm and rate:** Sinus rhythm, rate 68.
- **PR:** 0.16 **QRS:** 0.08 **QT:** 0.40.

- **Axis:** Normal. I and aVF are both positive.
- **BBB/HB:** None.
- **Hypertrophy:** None.
- **Miscellaneous effects:** None.
- **Infarction:** No evidence of ischemia or infarction.

5.

- **Rhythm and rate:** Sinus tachycardia, rate 150.
- **PR:** 0.14 **QRS:** 0.06 **QT:** 0.24.
- **Axis:** Normal.
- **BB/HB:** None.
- **Hypertrophy:** None. In fact, the voltage is pretty low throughout most leads.
- **Miscellaneous effects:** None.
- **Infarction:** No evidence of ischemia or infarction. Those are not Q waves in V_1 to V_2, in case you thought it was an anteroseptal MI. There's a teeny R wave there.

6.

- **Rhythm and rate:** Sinus rhythm, rate 71.
- **PR:** 0.20 **QRS:** 0.12 **QT:** 0.40.
- **Axis:** Left axis deviation. Lead I is positive and aVF is negative.
- **BBB/HB:** LBBB.
- **Hypertrophy:** None.
- **Miscellaneous effects:** None.
- **Infarction:** No evidence of ischemia or infarction.

7.

- **Rhythm and rate:** Atrial flutter with 2:1 conduction? Atrial rate 250, ventricular rate 115.
- **PR:** 0.16 **QRS:** 0.10 **QT:** 0.28.
- **Axis:** Left axis deviation. Lead I is positive and aVF is negative.
- **BBB/HB:** None.
- **Hypertrophy:** LVH by voltage criteria.
- **Miscellaneous effects:** No miscellaneous effects. The incredibly tall, pointy T wave in V_3 is related to the huge QRS voltage in that lead.
- **Infarction:** Anteroseptal and inferior wall MI. Note the ST segment elevation in II, III, aVF, and V_1 to V_4. There are already significant Q waves in V_1 to V_3. This is a massive MI.

8.

- **Rhythm and rate:** Sinus rhythm, rate 75.
- **PR:** 0.18 **QRS:** 0.13 **QT:** 0.42.
- **Axis:** Left axis deviation. Lead I is positive and aVF is negative.
- **BBB/HB:** RBBB.
- **Hypertrophy:** None by our voltage criteria.
- **Miscellaneous effects:** None.
- **Infarction:** Probable old anteroseptal MI, as there is a loss of the normal small R wave in V_1 to V_2.

9.

- **Rhythm and rate:** Sinus rhythm, rate 65.
- **PR:** 0.18 **QRS:** 0.06 **QT:** 0.36.
- **Axis:** Normal. Leads I and aVF are both positive.
- **BBB/HB:** None.
- **Hypertrophy:** LVH. The S wave in V_2 is 11; the R wave in V_5 is 26. Total is 37.
- **Miscellaneous effects:** None.
- **Infarction:** Probable early repolarization. Note the very slight concave ST elevation in II, III, aVF, and V_3 to V_5. It would help to know the age of this patient and the symptoms (if any) to identify this with a higher probability of accuracy.

10.

- **Rhythm and rate:** Atrial flutter with 2:1 conduction. No way, you say? Look at V_1. See the teeny spike in the ST segment? That's a flutter wave. There's another one before the QRS. If the gain had been turned up higher, this would have been much more obvious. Atrial rate is about 250; ventricular rate is 125.
- **PR:** Not applicable **QRS:** 0.06 **QT:** 0.24.
- **Axis:** Left axis deviation. Lead I is positive and aVF is negative.
- **BBB/HB:** *Maybe* a LAHB, but not sure we can really say there's a Q wave in Lead I.
- **Hypertrophy:** None. In fact, the voltage is rather low in the frontal leads.
- **Miscellaneous effects:** None.
- **Infarction:** Acute anterior-septal-lateral MI. Note the ST elevation in V_1 to V_6. There are significant Q waves in V_1 to V_5. There is also *very slight* ST coving in III and aVF, so there may also be an inferior MI starting up.

11.

- **Rhythm and rate:** Sinus tachycardia, rate 101.
- **PR:** 0.12 **QRS:** 0.06 **QT:** 0.32.
- **Axis:** Left axis deviation. Lead I is positive and aVF is negative.
- **BBB/HB:** None.
- **Hypertrophy:** None.
- **Miscellaneous effects:** None.
- **Infarction:** Old inferior MI and old anterior MI. Note the significant Q waves in Leads III and aVF and also in V_2 to V_3. Also note the poor R wave progression. The transition zone is V_5 and should be around V_3 to V_4.

12.

- **Rhythm and rate:** Sinus rhythm, rate 60.
- **PR:** 0.20 **QRS:** 0.14 **QT:** 0.46.
- **Axis:** Left axis deviation. Lead I is positive and aVF is negative.
- **BBB/HB:** RBBB and LAHB. There is a QR configuration in V_1.
- **Hypertrophy:** None.
- **Miscellaneous effects:** None.
- **Infarction:** Acute anterior-septal-lateral MI. Note the ST elevation in V_1 to V_5. There are significant Q waves in V_1 to V_3.

13.

- **Rhythm and rate:** Sinus rhythm, rate 75.
- **PR:** 0.12 **QRS:** 0.14 **QT:** 0.42.
- **Axis:** Normal.
- **BBB/HB:** LBBB. Note the *huge* QS wave in V_1.
- **Hypertrophy:** None.
- **Miscellaneous effects:** None.
- **Infarction:** None.

14.

- **Rhythm and rate:** Sinus rhythm, rate 83.
- **PR:** 0.14 **QRS:** 0.08 **QT:** 0.34.
- **Axis:** Normal.
- **BBB/HB:** None.
- **Hypertrophy:** None.
- **Miscellaneous effects:** None.
- **Infarction:** Acute inferior MI. Note the ST elevation in II, III, and aVF, along with reciprocal ST depression in I, aVL, and V_2 to V_6.

15.

- **Rhythm and rate:** Atrial fibrillation with uncontrolled ventricular response.
- **PR:** Not applicable **QRS:** 0.04 **QT:** 0.16.
- **Axis:** Normal.
- **BBB/HB:** None.
- **Hypertrophy:** None. In fact, the voltage is rather low in the frontal leads.
- **Miscellaneous effects:** Digitalis effect? ST segments look a bit scooped in Leads II and V_6. This may be simply from the rapid heart rate, however.
- **Infarction:** None. There are widespread inverted T waves, but this isn't a surprise, given the heart rate. Some ischemia may be occurring.

16.

- **Rhythm and rate:** Atrial fibrillation, rate 100 to150, mean rate 130.
- **PR:** Not applicable **QRS:** 0.06 **QT:** 0.28.
- **Axis:** Normal.
- **BBB/HB:** None.
- **Hypertrophy:** None. In fact, the voltage is rather low in the frontal leads.
- **Miscellaneous effects:** None.
- **Infarction:** None.

17.

- **Rhythm and rate:** Sinus rhythm, rate 75.
- **PR:** 0.16 **QRS:** 0.14 **QT:** 0.40.
- **Axis:** Left axis deviation. Lead I is slightly more positive than negative and aVF is slightly more negative than positive.
- **BBB/HB:** RBBB and LAHB.
- **Hypertrophy:** None.
- **Miscellaneous effects:** None.
- **Infarction:** Acute anterior MI. Note the ST elevation in V_2 to V_4.

18.

- **Rhythm and rate:** Sinus rhythm, rate 94.
- **PR:** 0.16 **QRS:** 0.10 **QT:** 0.36.
- **Axis:** Normal. The aVF's QRS has a little blip downward and then is positive.
- **BBB/HB:** None.

- **Hypertrophy:** None.
- **Miscellaneous effects:** None.
- **Infarction:** Acute inferior-lateral MI. Note the ST elevation in II, III, aVF, and V_5 to V_6. V_5 to V_6 is much shallower elevation than II, III, and aVF, so you might miss it at first. But do you see it now?

19.

- **Rhythm and rate:** Sinus rhythm, rate 88, with one PVC.
- **PR:** 0.12 **QRS:** 0.08 **QT:** 0.32.
- **Axis:** Left axis deviation. Lead I is positive, and aVF is negative.
- **BBB/HB:** None.
- **Hypertrophy:** None. In fact, the voltage is rather low in the frontal leads.
- **Miscellaneous effects:** None.
- **Infarction:** None.

20.

- **Rhythm and rate:** Sinus rhythm, rate 65.
- **PR:** 0.16 **QRS:** 0.06 **QT:** 0.36.
- **Axis:** Normal.
- **BBB/HB:** None.
- **Hypertrophy:** None.
- **Miscellaneous effects:** None.
- **Infarction:** None.

CHAPTER FOUR
DDD versus VVI Practice

1. **Cannot tell which kind of pacemaker.** Because there are no paced beats at all, it is not possible to tell if it's a DDD or a VVI pacemaker.
2. **VVI.** There are pacemaker spikes preceding the QRS complexes, and there are no P waves in sight. Had this been a DDD pacemaker, there should have been some paced P waves also.
3. **DDD.** There are pacemaker spikes preceding the P waves and the QRS complexes.
4. **VVI.** There are four intrinsic beats and two paced beats on the strip. The paced beats pace only the ventricle. With this long a pause before a paced beat kicks in, a DDD pacemaker would have provided a paced P wave as well.

5. **DDD.** This strip has a little of everything. The first beat is all intrinsic. The second beat paces atrium and ventricle, as evidenced by the pacemaker spikes preceding the P wave and the QRS. The third beat has a paced P wave and an intrinsic QRS. The fourth, sixth, and seventh beats are all intrinsic. The fifth beat has an intrinsic P wave followed by a paced QRS.

Pacemaker Malfunctions Practice

1. **Undersensing and loss of capture.** We have pacemaker spikes in inappropriate places, such as inside the first QRS complex. It is clear this pacemaker is not sensing the QRS complexes, because it does nothing in response to those intrinsic complexes. The pacemaker should have been inhibited by the patient's intrinsic QRS complexes. Also note the spikes are regular at a rate of 60. This is essentially a fixed-rate pacemaker now because it's not sensing anything. In addition, there is loss of capture, as evidenced by the pacemaker spikes not followed by Ps or QRSs at times when they should have been. The patient's underlying rhythm is idioventricular rhythm with a rate of 23.

2. **No malfunction at this time.** This strip shows a normally functioning DDD pacemaker. Note the upward atrial spikes followed by a tiny blip of a P wave, then a ventricular spike followed by a wide QRS. Although the pacemaker seems fine right now, it could be that it malfunctions intermittently, causing the symptoms, so the patient will still need close observation. It is also possible that the patient's dizziness and syncope were caused by something totally unrelated to the pacemaker.

3. **No malfunction noted.** This strip shows a normally functioning DDD pacemaker. See the small intrinsic P waves preceding each QRS? The pacemaker senses them and tracks them, providing the paced QRS to follow those Ps because the patient does not have her own QRS complexes in the programmed time.

4. **Failure to fire.** There are two intrinsic P waves on this strip. The pacemaker should have sensed them and provided a paced QRS to follow them. In addition, it should have paced the atrium and then the ventricle, as necessary, at its programmed rate of 70. It didn't. There's not a pacemaker spike in sight.

5. **No malfunction noted.** The pacemaker rate is set at 60, and it fires at 60 when the atrial fibrillation slows down. Note the pacing interval from spike to spike on the three paced beats. Now look at the interval between the second QRS and the paced beat that follows. It's exactly the same interval. The pacemaker is, therefore, sensing the underlying rhythm, and it's firing and capturing appropriately.

Practice Quiz

1. Digitalis is classified as a **cardiac glycoside.**
2. Class I antiarrhythmic medications **affect phase 0 of the action potential by blocking the influx of sodium into the cardiac cell.**
3. Atropine **increases the heart rate.**
4. Vasoconstriction **causes the blood pressure to increase.**
5. **True.** The AED is meant for use by the lay public.
6. Class III antiarrhythmic medications **affect phase 3 of the action potential. They interfere with the movement of potassium into the cardiac cell during repolarization.**
7. **Therapeutic hypothermia is used in post–cardiac arrest patients who regain spontaneous circulation. Their body temperature is lowered to 90 to 93 degrees in order to decrease ischemia, particularly of the brain, that can result from the cardiac arrest.**
8. The 3 letters of the pacemaker code refer to **the chamber paced, the chamber sensed,** and **the response to sensed events.**
9. Cardioversion differs from defibrillation in that **cardioversion is synchronized with the cardiac cycle; defibrillation is not synchronized.**
10. Antitachycardia pacing is used to **slow the heart rate—to abort a tachycardia. The pacemaker fires out a series of rapid electrical impulses to interrupt the tachycardia's circuit, thereby stopping that rhythm.** Pacing for bradycardia **involves sending out an electrical impulse to increase the heart rate.**

Critical Thinking Exercises

1. a. Atrial Fibrillation—**cardiovert.**
   b. V-tach with pulse—**cardiovert.**
   c. V-fib—**defibrillate.**
   d. V-tach without pulse—**defibrillate.**
   e. SVT—**cardiovert.**
2. a. The rhythm **is atrial flutter with two flutter waves to each QRS.** Heart rate is 150.
   b. **The pacemaker is doing nothing** that we can see. We have to assume it is sensing the patient's own rhythm and knows it doesn't need to fire.

c. Because the patient has a temporary pacemaker in place and therefore has the pulse generator at the bedside in easy reach, **we can use the pacemaker to overdrive this rhythm and slow the heart rate.**

d. The rhythm is **atrial fibrillation; heart rate mean is 40; range is 19 to 71.**

e. **The pacemaker is doing nothing.** It's set at a rate of 60 so it shouldn't let the heart rate drop below that.

f. There is indeed a pacer malfunction—it's **failure to fire.**

g. **The battery may need to be changed or the pacer wire or cable may need to be changed.**

h. With the first rhythm, the **heart rate is very rapid, causing decreased time for the ventricles to fill with blood.** Less blood goes in, so less blood is pumped out to the body. With the second rhythm, the **heart rate is very slow. Unless the heart is able to compensate for the decreased heart rate by increasing the amount of blood pumped out with each beat, cardiac output will fall.** Both rhythms can, therefore, result in Mr. Johnson's low blood pressure and feeling of faintness.

3. a. The symptoms are caused by his use of nitroglycerine and sildenafil together. Sildenafil must not be used with nitrate medications as they can cause a dangerous drop in blood pressure. With a low blood pressure, the heart does not receive adequate blood flow—it can become ischemic and can infarct.

   b. Teach Mr. Lohtrip about the proper use of his medications.

CHAPTER FIVE
Scenario A: Mr. Johnson

1. Of concern is the **ST segment elevation in Lead II** on this strip. The sinus bradycardia is not a concern, especially as Mr. Johnson had been asleep, but the ST elevation is worrisome.

2. **Mr. Johnson is having an inferior wall MI**, as evidenced by the ST elevation in Leads II, III, and aVF and by the reciprocal ST depression in the anterior leads.

3. **Nitroglycerin dilates coronary arteries and thus increases the flow to the tissues.**

4. **The oxygen will improve tissue concentration of oxygen and can help prevent arrhythmias and decrease the heart's workload.**

5. Thrombolytic medications **dissolve blood clots.**

6. The danger of giving thrombolytics to someone who had recent surgery is that **severe bleeding may occur at the surgical site.**

7. The rhythm is **ventricular tachycardia**. Heart rate is about 300.

8. **Potassium deficit (hypokalemia)** can cause V-tach.

9. **Hypoxia** is another blood abnormality that can cause V-tach.

10. **Amiodarone or lidocaine** could be used to abolish the V-tach.

11. **Morphine** is another medication that can be used to treat chest pain.

12. **The MI is extending into the lateral wall now**, as evidenced by the new ST elevation in Leads V_5 to V_6.

13. This rhythm is **2:1 AV block**. There are two P waves to every QRS on this strip.

14. This rhythm can **cause the cardiac output to drop**.

15. The nurse should now **give atropine** to speed up the heart rate until a transcutaneous pacemaker can be utilized.

16. The block could be at the **AV node or the bundle branches**.

17. If the block were at the bundle branches, **atropine may have no effect on the heart rate**. Atropine speeds up the rate of the sinus node and increases AV conduction, causing the impulses to come more rapidly. The impulses blast through the AV node only to arrive at the still-blocked bundle branches (atropine has no effect on the bundle branches). Epinephrine and/or pacing would be indicated for a block at the bundle branches.

18. This rhythm is **sinus rhythm**.

19. **Mr. Johnson should have no symptoms** from this rhythm. He should in fact feel much better now that his heart rate is more normal.

20. The two coronary arteries blocked were probably the **right coronary artery, which supplies the inferior wall of the left ventricle, and the circumflex, which supplies the lateral wall.**

Scenario B: Ms. Capitano

1. The rhythm is **SVT**. The heart rate is about 150, the rhythm is regular, and P waves are not discernible.

2. The likely cause of this rhythm in this case is **excessive caffeine intake**.

3. **The heart rate slowed dramatically to a junctional bradycardia.** This is not unusual after adenosine administration. In fact, sometimes the heart completely stops for a few seconds before the sinus node kicks back in.

4. **The tachycardia is dropping her cardiac output to dangerously low levels.**

Scenario C: Mr. Farley

1. The rhythm is **slow atrial fibrillation**. Note the wavy, undulating baseline and the absence of P waves.
2. **In atrial fibrillation, there is no atrial kick at all**, thus causing a drop in cardiac output of about 15% to 30%.
3. **Digitalis toxicity can cause almost any arrhythmia, such as junctional tachycardia, atrial tachycardia, sinus arrests, sinus blocks, all degrees of AV blocks, and slow junctional and ventricular rhythms.**
4. The rhythm is **asystole**.
5. **Epinephrine** would be appropriate to give, as it speeds up the heart rate and can help restore pumping function in cardiac arrest.
6. A pacemaker would **prevent Mr. Farley's heart rate from going too slow**.
7. Loss of capture is evidenced by the **pacemaker spikes not followed by a QRS complex**.
8. Capture might be restored by **repositioning Mr. Farley in bed or by increasing the voltage sent out by the pacemaker.**
9. A pacemaker provides the possibility of **overdriving the tachycardia**. The pacemaker rate is dialed up to a rate exceeding the patient's heart rate. The pacemaker then assumes control of (usurps) the underlying rhythm. The pacemaker can then be slowly turned down, allowing the sinus node to assume control.
10. **Amiodarone decreases the irritability of the ventricle and makes it less responsive to ventricular impulses.**
11. Mr. Farley should be instructed to **follow his physician's prescription, not to add or subtract doses on his own. If he does not feel well, he should contact his physician or go to the hospital ER.**

Scenario D: Mr. Lew

1. This EKG reveals that **Mr. Lew has suffered an extensive anterior MI**, as evidenced by the ST elevation in I, aVL, and all the precordial leads, along with reciprocal ST depression in the inferior leads.
2. This rhythm is **accelerated idioventricular rhythm**.
3. It usually requires **no treatment**. AIVR is usually well-tolerated.
4. **It was believed in the past that the occurrence of AIVR following use of thrombolytics was a sign of reperfusion of the myocardium**, but recent research has shown that not to be the case.
5. Mr. Lew has now **extended his MI into the inferior wall**, as evidenced by the new ST elevation in II, III, and aVF. This is a catastrophic development.
6. **The right coronary artery is also blocked**.
7. The ST depression in the first EKG was **a reciprocal change**.
8. The rhythm is **ventricular fibrillation**.
9. The rhythm is **agonal rhythm (dying heart)**.

Scenario E: Mrs. Epstein

1. The rhythm is **third-degree AV block**. Note that the P-P intervals are regular and the R-R intervals are also regular, but at a different rate. The PR intervals vary.
2. **Her pacemaker is doing nothing**. There are no pacemaker spikes anywhere.
3. The likely cause of this is a **dead pacemaker battery**.
4. The rhythm is **dual-chamber pacing**. Note the pacemaker spikes preceding the P waves and QRS complexes.
5. **The pacemaker is functioning properly**.

Scenario F: Mr. Calico

1. The rhythm is **asystole**. There is a flat line—no P waves, QRS complexes, or T waves.
2. **He would have no pulse, no breathing, no movement. His skin would be cool and ashen or cyanotic in color.**
3. Treatment would include **immediate CPR and administration of intravenous epinephrine**.
4. The rhythm is **SVT**, heart rate 150. This is a typical reaction to epinephrine—the heart rate speeds up dramatically.
5. There is an **anteroseptal MI**. Note the ST elevation in V_1 to V_4, with reciprocal ST depression in II, III, and aVF.
6. **The ST segment has returned to normal**, indicating the MI has been aborted.
7. **The problem was the nurse tried to cardiovert V-fib.** Cardioversion requires that the electrical shock to the heart be synchronized with the QRS complex. In V-fib there are no QRS complexes with which to synchronize, so the shock is never delivered. The nurse must change the machine setting to **defibrillate** (take it off synchronous mode) and try again.

Scenario G: Mrs. Taylor

1. **Hyperkalemia is elevated blood potassium level.** It can cause tall, pointy T waves and eventually wide QRS complexes. The EKG shows very wide QRS complexes.
2. The rhythm is **idioventricular rhythm**, rate about 28. Note the slow heart rate and the wide QRS complexes.
3. **The QRS complex has narrowed.**

Scenario H: Mr. Foster

1. The rhythm is **atrial fibrillation, heart rate 94 to 167, mean rate 120**.
2. The physician did not want to cardiovert Mr. Foster because **she didn't know how long he'd been in atrial fibrillation.** Cardioversion could send blood clots out of his atria into the coronary arteries, his brain arteries, or his pulmonary artery, causing MI, stroke, or pulmonary embolus.
3. It's a **STEMI**. There is ST segment elevation.
4. The MI is **extensive anterior**.
5. Cocaine can cause **coronary artery spasm**, which can occlude blood flow to the myocardium in a given area and can cause MIs.

Scenario I: Mr. Frye

1. The rhythm is **sinus rhythm for the first three beats, then changing to PAT.** The fourth beat is a PAC and so are the beats that follow. This "run of PACs" is called PAT.

2. The heart rate starts off **at 100 and then increases to about 187 once in PAT. Mean rate is 170.**
3. The **vagus nerve slows conduction through the AV node and slows the heart rate**.
4. The rhythm is **sinus rhythm with a border-line first-degree AV block. PR interval is 0.20 seconds.**
5. Adenosine can cause **a brief period of asystole.**
6. **No, that is not evident on this strip**.
7. Other treatments could include **beta-blockers, calcium channel blockers, digitalis,** and **electrical cardioversion.**

Scenario J: Mrs. Terry

1. The rhythm is **sinus rhythm with first-degree AV block (PR interval about 0.22 seconds), heart rate 100.**
2. There is **ST segment elevation.**
3. The EKG shows **ST elevation in Leads II, III, and aVF along with reciprocal ST depression in Leads I, aVL, and V_1 to V_5. There's a tiny bit of ST elevation in V_6. Thus there is an inferior MI (II, III, and aVF) with perhaps lateral wall involvement (V_6).**
4. The preferred treatment for this acute MI is **PCI.**
5. The suspected involved coronary artery would be the **left anterior descending** (with maybe a bit starting up in the circumflex, causing that little ST elevation in V_6).

Glossary

Absolute refractory period: The period in which the cardiac cell will not respond to any stimulus, no matter how strong.

Acetylcholine: A hormone released as a result of parasympathetic stimulation.

Action potential: The depolarization and repolarization events that take place at the cell membrane. Also refers to the diagram associated with these polarity events.

Acute: Newly occurring.

AED: A defibrillator meant for use by the lay public.

Age indeterminate: A recent ST elevation MI, but can't be sure of the MI's exact age.

Agonal rhythm: A ventricular rhythm characterized by slow, irregular QRS complexes and absent P waves. Also called *dying heart.*

AICD: Automated implantable cardioverter-defibrillator. An implanted device that shocks the heart out of certain dangerous rhythms, such as V-Tach.

Algorithm: A flowchart.

Amplifier: An instrument that magnifies a signal.

Amplitude: The height of the waves and complexes on the EKG.

Angina: Chest pain caused by a decrease in myocardial blood flow.

Anginal equivalent: An individual's version of chest pain. May not involve pain at all—could be shortness of breath, fatigue, or other symptoms.

Angiogram: An invasive procedure in which dye is injected into blood vessels in order to determine their patency (openness).

Antegrade: In a forward direction.

Anterior axillary line: An imaginary line down from the front of the axilla (armpit).

Anterior STEMI: ST elevation MI affecting the anterior wall of the left ventricle.

Anterior wall: The front side of the left ventricle.

Anteroseptal: Pertaining to the anterior and septal walls of the left ventricle.

Anteroseptal STEMI: ST elevation MI affecting the septum and part or all of the anterior wall of the left ventricle.

Antiarrhythmic: Medications used to treat or prevent arrhythmias.

Anticoagulants: Medications used to prevent blood clot formation.

Antihypertensives: Medications used to treat hypertension.

Antitachycardia pacing: A special pacemaker function that interrupts tachycardias and helps convert the rhythm back to sinus rhythm.

Aorta: Largest artery in the body, into which the left ventricle empties.

Aortic stenosis: Narrowed opening to the aortic valve.

Aortic valve: Valve located between the left ventricle and aorta.

Apex: The pointy part of the heart where it rests on the diaphragm.

Arrhythmia: Abnormal heart rhythm.

Arteriole: A small artery that empties into a capillary bed.

Artery: A blood vessel that carries blood away from the heart to the tissues or the lungs.

Artifact: Unwanted jitter or interference on the EKG tracing.

Asystole: No heart beat. Characterized by a flat line on the EKG.

Atrial kick: The phase of diastole in which the atria contract to propel their blood into the ventricles.

Atrial rate: The heart rate of the P waves (or P wave alternatives such as flutter waves).

Atrial tissue: Tissue in the atria.

Atrioventricular block: Also called AV block. A block in impulse transmission from atrium to ventricle.

Atrioventricular valves: Also called AV valves. Heart valves located between atrium and ventricle.

Atrium: The upper, thin-walled receiving chambers of the heart.

Augment: Increase.

Augmented leads: Leads in which the EKG machine must increase (augment) the size of the waves and complexes. Includes aVR, aVL, and aVF.

Automated implantable cardioverter-defibrillator (AICD): See AICD.

Automaticity: The ability of cardiac cells to initiate an impulse without outside stimulation.

Autonomic nervous system: The nervous system controlling involuntary biological functions.

AV blocks (atrioventricular blocks): Disturbances in conduction in which some or all impulses from the sinus node are either delayed on their trip to the ventricles or do not reach the ventricle at all.

AV dissociation (atrioventricular dissociation): A condition in which the atria and ventricles depolarize and contract independently of each other.

AV interval: The interval between atrial and ventricular pacemaker spikes (It's an electronic PR interval).

AV junction (atrioventricular junction): Conductive tissue between the AV node and the atria.

AV node (atrioventricular node): The group of specialized cells in the conduction system that slows impulse transmission to allow atrial contraction to occur.

Axillary: Referring to the armpit.

Axis: The mean direction of the heart's current flow.

Axis circle: A circle that is formed by joining the ends of lead lines I, II, III, aVR, aVL, and aVF. This makes calculation of the electrical axis possible.

Axis deviation: An abnormal axis.

Base: The top of the heart; the area from which the great vessels emerge.

Baseline: The line from which the EKG waves and complexes take off. Also called the isoelectric line.

Bayes's theorem: The theorem that states that the predictive value of a test is based not only on the accuracy of the test itself but on the patient's probability of disease, as determined by a risk assessment done prior to the testing.

Beta-blockers: Class of cardiac medications that slows the heart rate, decreases blood pressure, and reduces cardiac workload.

Beta-receptors: Receptors that affect heart rate, contractility, and airway size.

Bifascicular block: A block of both fascicles of the left bundle branch, or a right bundle branch block plus a hemiblock.

Bigeminy: Every other beat is an abnormal beat.

Bipolar: Having a positive and a negative pole.

Blood pressure: The pressure exerted on the arterial walls by the circulating blood.

Bradyarrhythmia: An arrhythmia with a heart rate less than 60.

Bradycardia: Slow heart rate, usually less than 60.

Bronchodilators: Medications that dilate constricted airway passages in individuals with asthma, bronchitis, or emphysema.

Bundle branch block: A block in conduction through one of the bundle branches.

Bundle branches: Conduction pathways extending from the bundle of His in the lower right atrium to the Purkinje fibers in the ventricles. There is a right and a left bundle branch.

Bundle of His: A confluence of conduction fibers between the AV node and the bundle branches.

Capillary bed: The smallest blood vessels in the body; where nutrient and gas exchange occurs.

Capture: The depolarization of the atrium and/or ventricle as a result of a pacemaker's firing. Determined by the presence of a P wave and/or QRS after the pacemaker spike.

Cardiac arrest: An emergency in which the heart stops beating.

Cardiac cycle: The mechanical events that occur to pump blood. Consists of diastole and systole.

Cardiac output: The amount of blood expelled by the heart each minute. Measured as heart rate times stroke volume.

Cardiogenic shock: Shock induced by heart failure.

Cardiologist: A physician specializing in cardiac disease.

Cardioversion: Synchronized electrical shock to the heart to convert an abnormal rhythm back to sinus rhythm.

Carotid sinus massage: A method of slowing the heart rate by rubbing on the carotid artery in the neck.

Catheter ablation: A procedure in which a catheter is utilized to destroy the irritable heart tissue responsible for causing an arrhythmia.

Chart speed: EKG machine feature that regulates the speed of the paper printout.

Chordae tendineae: Tendinous cords that attach to the AV valves and prevent them from everting.

Chronotropic incompetence: Inability of the heart rate to increase with stress.

Chronotropic reserve: The ability of the heart rate to increase with exercise.

Circumflex coronary artery: The branch off the left main coronary artery that feeds oxygenated blood to the lateral wall of the left ventricle.

Clockwise: Moving in the direction of clock hands.

Code: Cardiac arrest.

Complete compensatory pause: Normally follows PVCs. Measures two R-R cycles from the beat preceding the PVC to the beat following the PVC.

Conduction system: A network of specialized cells whose job is to create and conduct the electrical impulses that control the cardiac cycle.

Conduction system cells: Cardiac cells whose job is to create and conduct electrical signals to trigger a heartbeat.

Conductivity: The ability of a cardiac cell to pass an impulse along to neighboring cells.

Congestive heart failure (CHF): Fluid buildup in the lungs as a result of the heart's inability to pump adequately.

Contractile cells: Cardiac cells whose job is to contract and cause blood to flow.

Contractility: The ability of a cardiac cell to contract and do work.

Contraindications: Reasons to avoid doing a test or procedure.

Coronary arteries: The arteries that feed oxygenated blood to the myocardium.

Coronary vein: Vein that returns deoxygenated blood from the heart tissues back to the right atrium.

Counterclockwise: In a direction opposite the way the clock hands move.

Couplet: A pair of beats.

Coved ST segment: Rounded ST segment elevation typical of an STEMI. Also called convex ST segment elevation.

CPK: Creatine phosphokinase. Chemical released by the heart during an MI.

Critical rate: The rate at which a bundle branch block appears or disappears.

Decreased cardiac output: Inadequate blood flow to meet the body's needs.

Decreased diastolic filling time: Caused by tachycardias. The decreased time between beats for the heart to fill up with blood.

Defibrillation: Asynchronous electrical shock to the heart, used to treat ventricular fibrillation and pulseless V-tach.

Delta wave: A slurred upstroke to the QRS complex, seen in Wolff-Parkinson-White Syndrome.

Depolarization: The wave of electrical current that changes the resting negatively charged cardiac cell to a positively charged one.

Diaphoresis: Sweating, usually a cold sweat. Also referred to as "cold and clammy."

Diastasis: The phase in diastole in which the atrial and ventricular pressures are equalizing.

Diastole: The phase of the cardiac cycle in which the ventricles fill with blood.

Digital converter: A device in an EKG machine that converts an analog signal to a digital one.

Digitalis toxicity: Overabundance of the medication digitalis in the bloodstream.

Dissecting aneurysm: The ballooning out of an artery into the wall of the artery itself.

Dissociation: The lack of relationship between two pacemaker sites in the heart.

Diuretics: Medications given to increase the urine output.

Early repolarization: Phases 1 and 2 of the action potential.

Ectopic rhythms: Rhythms originating in any pacemaker other than the sinus node.

Einthoven's law: The height of the QRS complexes in Lead I +Lead III = Lead II.

Einthoven's triangle: The triangle formed by joining Leads I, II, and III at the ends.

Electrocardiogram: The physical printout of the electrical signals generated by the heart.

Electrocardiography: The process of recording the heart's electrical signals.

Electrodes: Adhesive patches attached to the skin to receive the electrical signals from the heart.

Electrolytes: Blood chemicals.

Embolus: Blood clot that has broken off and is traveling through a blood vessel.

Endocardium: The innermost layer of the heart.

Epicardium: Outer layer of the heart.

Erectile dysfunction medications: Medications that treat erectile problems in males.

Ergometer: An arm bicycle used in stress testing.

Escape: A safety mechanism in which a lower pacemaker fires at its slower inherent rate when the faster, predominant pacemaker fails.

Escaping: A lower pacemaker taking over when a higher pacemaker fails.

Event monitor: A small device that can be used to determine if sporadic arrhythmias or ischemia are present.

Evolution: The gradual EKG changes that occur in an acute ST elevation MI.

Excitability: The ability of a cardiac cell to depolarize when stimulated.

Extensive anterior STEMI: A large ST elevation MI affecting the anterior and lateral walls of the left ventricle.

Fascicle: A branch.

Fibrillation: The wiggling or twitching of the atrium or ventricle.

Firing: The pacemaker's generation of an electrical impulse.

Fixed-rate pacemaker: An old-fashioned pacemaker that paced at a programmed rate with no regard to the patient's own intrinsic rhythm or beats.

Foci: Locations.

Focus: Location.

Frontal leads: Limb Leads I, II, III, aVR, aVL, and aVF. Leads located on the front of the body.

Fusion beats: A combination of a sinus beat and a PVC. Shape is intermediate between that of the sinus beat and the PVC.

Gain: EKG machine feature that regulates the height of the waves and complexes.

Glaucoma medications: Medications that decrease the eyeball pressure.

Glottis: The flap over the top of the windpipe.

Heart rate: The number of times the heart beats in one minute.

Heart rhythm: A pattern of successive heart beats.

Hemiblock: A block of one of the left bundle branch's fascicles.

Hexiaxial diagram: A diagram of the six frontal leads intersecting at the center; serves as the basis for the axis circle.

Holter monitor: A device used for 24-hour cardiac monitoring to check for arrhythmias or ST segment abnormalities.

Hyperacute changes: Those seen in the earliest stages of a disease or condition.

Hypercalcemia: Elevated blood calcium level.

Hyperkalemia: Elevated blood potassium level.

Hypertension: High blood pressure.

Hypertrophic cardiomyopathy: Heart disease caused by an overgrowth of the interventricular septum.

Hypertrophy: Overgrowth of myocardial tissue.

Hyperventilating: Breathing very rapidly.

Hypocalcemia: Low blood calcium level.

Hypokalemia: Low blood potassium level.

Hypotension: Low blood pressure.

Hypoxia: Low blood oxygen level.

Indeterminate axis: An axis that is between −90 and +−180 degrees.

Indications: Reasons to perform a test or procedure.

Indicative changes: EKG changes that indicate the presence of an MI.

Infarction: Death of tissue. A myocardial infarction (MI) is a heart attack.

Inferior STEMI: ST elevation MI involving the inferior wall of the left ventricle.

Inferior vena cava (IVC):   Large vein that returns deoxygenated blood to the right atrium from the lower chest, abdomen, and legs.

Inferior wall: The bottom wall of the left ventricle.

Inherent: Preset.

Injury: Damage to tissue.

Inotropic incompetence: The inability of the blood pressure to increase with exercise.

Inotropic reserve: The ability of the blood pressure to increase with exercise.

Interatrial septum: The muscular band of tissue separating the right and left atria.

Interatrial tracts: The pathways that carry the electrical impulse from the sinus node through the atrial tissue.

Intercostal spaces: Spaces between the ribs.

Internodal tracts: Pathways that carry electrical impulses from the sinus node to the AV node.

Intervals: Measurements of time between EKG waves and complexes.

Interventricular septum: The muscular band of tissue separating right and left ventricles.

Intrinsic: The patient's own. Intrinsic beats are the patient's own beats.

Inverted: Upside down.

Ions: Electrically charged particles.

Irritability: Also called usurpation. The cardiac cell fires in prematurely, taking control away from the predominant pacemaker.

Ischemia: Oxygen deprivation in the tissues.

Isoelectric: As much above the baseline as below.

Isoelectric line: The flat line between the EKG waves and complexes. Also called the baseline.

Isovolumetric: Maintaining the same volume.

Isovolumetric contraction: The first phase of systole. The ventricles are contracting but no blood flow is occurring because all the valves are still closed.

Isovolumetric relaxation: The final phase of systole. The semilunar valves slam shut and blood flow from the ventricles stops.

J point: The point where the QRS complex and ST segment join together.

Kent bundle: The accessory pathway in WPW.

Late potentials: Electrical potentials that occur late in the QRS complex and can be a sign of ventricular irritability and impending ventricular arrhythmias.

Lateral wall: The left side wall of the left ventricle.

Lateral wall STEMI: ST elevation MI affecting the lateral wall of the left ventricle.

Lead: An electrocardiographic picture of the heart.

Lead wires: Wires that attach the electrode patches to the EKG machine.

Leakage current: Small amount of electrical current that escapes from an implanted device such as a pacemaker.

Left anterior descending coronary artery: A branch of the left main coronary artery. It feeds oxygenated blood to the anterior wall of the left ventricle.

Left anterior hemiblock: Block of the left anterior fascicle of the left bundle branch.

Left axis deviation: An axis between 0 and −90 degrees.

Left bundle branch: Conduction fibers that carry the cardiac impulses down the left side of the septum to the left ventricle.

Left common bundle branch: The part of the left bundle branch before it divides into its fascicles.

Left main coronary artery: The coronary artery that branches off into the circumflex and left anterior descending coronary arteries.

Left posterior hemiblock: Block of the left posterior fascicle of the left bundle branch.

Limb leads: Leads attached to the limbs. Includes I, II, III, aVR, aVL, and aVF.

Low cardiac output: Inadequate amount of blood pumped out by the heart every minute.

Macroshock: A large electrical shock caused by improper or faulty grounding of electrical equipment.

Mean rate (mean heart rate):   The average heart rate.

Mediastinum: The cavity between the lungs, in which the heart is located.

MET: Metabolic equivalent, a measurement of oxygen consumption.

Microshock: A small electrical shock made possible by a conduit, such as a pacemaker, directly in the heart.

Midaxillary line: An imaginary line down from the middle of the axilla (armpit).

Midclavicular line: An imaginary line down from the middle of the clavicle (collarbone).

Mitral: Valve that separates the left atrium and left ventricle.

Multifocal: Coming from more than one location.

Myocardial infarction: Heart attack.

Myocardium: The muscular layer of the heart.

Necroses: Dies.

Neuropathy: Condition that causes a decrease in sensation, especially pain, in susceptible individuals.

Nitrates: Medications used to dilate coronary arteries and improve coronary blood flow.

Nonconducted PAC: A premature P wave not followed by a QRS complex.

Norepinephrine: The chemical released by the adrenal gland when stimulated by the sympathetic nervous system.

Normal axis: Axis between 0 and +90 degrees.

NSTEMI: Non-ST elevation MI.

Occlusion: Blockage.

Oversensed: Pacemaker sensed something it shouldn't have, such as a beat from another chamber.

Oxygen: An element inhaled from the atmosphere that is necessary for body function.

Pacemaker: The intrinsic or artificial focus that propagates or initiates the cardiac impulse.

Pacing interval: The programmed interval between paced beats.

Papillary muscle: The muscle to which the chordae tendineae are attached at the bottom.

Parasympathetic nervous system: The division of the autonomic nervous system that slows the heart rate, lowers blood pressure, stimulates digestion, and constricts pupils—all signs of the "rest-and-digest" response.

Paroxysmal: Occurring suddenly and stopping just as suddenly.

PCI: Percutaneous coronary intervention. A balloon procedure to open a blocked coronary artery.

Perfusing: Supplying blood to.

Perfusion: The supplying of blood and nutrients to tissues.

Pericardial fluid: Small amount of fluid found between the layers of the pericardial sac.

Pericarditis: An inflammation of the pericardium.

Pericardium: The sac that encloses the heart.

Plateau phase: The phase of the action potential in which the waveform levels off (flattens out). Phase 2 is the plateau phase.

Platelet aggregation: Clumping of platelets to form clots to stop bleeding.

Platelets: Cells responsible for blood clotting.

Polarized: Possessing an electrical charge.

Polymorphic: Possessing multiple shapes.

Postangioplasty evaluation: Evaluation of the patient's condition following a procedure to open up blocked coronary arteries.

Posterior descending artery: A branch off the right coronary artery that provides blood flow to the posterior wall of the left ventricle.

Posterior MI: MI affecting the posterior wall of the left ventricle.

Posterior wall: The back wall of the left ventricle.

P-P interval: The distance (interval) between consecutive P waves.

Precordial: Pertaining to the chest.

Precordial leads: The six leads on the chest (V1 through V6).

Pre-excitation: Depolarizing tissue earlier than normal.

PR interval: Measurement of time it takes the cardiac impulse to travel from atrium to ventricle.

Protodiastole: The phase of systole in which the blood flow out of the ventricles slows because of equalizing pressures between the ventricles and the aorta and pulmonary artery.

PR segment: Flat line between the P wave and the QRS complex.

Pulmonary artery: Large artery that takes deoxygenated blood from the right ventricle to the lungs. It is the ONLY artery that carries deoxygenated blood.

Pulmonary embolus: Blood clot in the lung.

Pulmonary veins: Four veins that return oxygenated blood from the lungs to the left atrium. They are the ONLY veins that carry oxygenated blood.

Pulmonic valve: Valve located between the right ventricle and the pulmonary artery.

Purkinje fibers: Fibers at the terminal ends of the bundle branches. Responsible for transmitting the impulses into the ventricular myocardium.

P wave: The EKG wave reflecting atrial depolarization.

P wave asystole: A type of asystole that still has P waves.

QRS complex: The EKG complex representing ventricular depolarization.

QRS interval: The spiked wave on the EKG. Represents ventricular depolarization.

QS wave: A QRS complex with only a downward wave—no upward wave(s).

QT interval: Measures ventricular depolarization and repolarization time.

Quadrigeminy: Every fourth beat is abnormal.

Q wave: A downward wave preceding an R wave in the QRS complex. If a Q wave is present, it is ALWAYS the first wave of the QRS complex.

R′   Pronounced "R prime." Is the second R wave in a QRS complex.

Rapid-filling phase: The first phase of diastole in which the ventricles rapidly fill with blood from the atria.

Rapid repolarization: Phase 3 of the action potential.

Rate-related bundle branch blocks: Bundle branch blocks that appear only at certain heart rates.

Reciprocal changes: EKG changes (ST depression) seen in the area electrically opposite the infarcted area.

Refractory: Resistant to.

Regularity: Spacing of the P waves or QRS complexes.

Relative refractory period: The period in which only a strong stimulus will cause depolarization of the cardiac cell.

Reperfusion arrhythmia: A rhythm, usually AIVR, that was thought to result from the return of blood and oxygen supply to tissues that have been deprived for a period of time.

Repolarization: The wave of electrical current that returns the cardiac cell to its resting, electrically negative state.

Resuscitation: Restoring respirations and/or pulse by way of artificial respiration and cardiac compressions.

Retrograde: In a backward direction.

Rhythm strip: A printout of one or two leads at a time, done on special rolls of paper.

Right axis deviation: An axis between +90 to +−80 degrees.

Right bundle branch: Conduction fibers that carry the cardiac impulses down the right side of the septum to the right ventricle.

Right coronary artery (RCA):   The coronary artery that feeds oxygenated blood to the right ventricle and the inferior wall of the left ventricle.

R-on-T phenomenon: The PVC that falls on the T wave of the preceding beat. Predisposes to rapid arrhythmias.

R-R interval: The distance (interval) between consecutive QRS complexes. Usually measured at the peaks of the R waves.

R wave: An upward wave in the QRS complex.

Scooping ST segment: Rounded ST segment seen with digitalis effect.

Segment: The flat line between EKG waves and complexes.

Semilunar valves: Half-moon-shaped. Refers to the aortic and pulmonic valves.

Sensing: The ability of an artificial pacemaker to "see" the intrinsic rhythm in order to determine whether the pacemaker needs to fire.

Sensitivity: The ability of a test to pick out the people who are truly diseased.

Septum: The fibrous tissue that separates the heart into right and left sides.

Sinus node: The normal pacemaker of the heart.

Sleep apnea: Temporary, often repetitive cessation of breathing during sleep.

Sodium-potassium pump: The active transport system that returns the cardiac cell to its resting, electrically negative state following depolarization.

Somatic: Referring to the body.

Specificity: The ability of a test to exclude those who are not diseased.

STEMI: ST elevation MI.

Stenosis: Narrowed opening.

Stenotic: Pertaining to stenosis.

Stent: A wire mesh inserted into a coronary artery to hold it open following PCI.

Sternum: Breastbone.

Stress test: A test done to determine the presence of coronary artery disease. Can be done using exercise or medications to stress the heart.

Stress testing: A method of utilizing a bicycle or treadmill to stress the heart and determine if coronary disease is present.

ST segment: The flat line between the QRS complex and the T wave.

Subendocardial: Referring to the myocardial layer just beneath the endocardium.

Submaximal test: A stress test that is concluded when 70% of the target heart rate is reached.

Superior vena cava (SVC):   Large vein that returns deoxygenated blood to the right atrium from the head, neck, upper chest, and arms.

Supernormal period: The period in which the cardiac cell is "hyper" and will respond to a very weak stimulus.

Supine: Back-lying.

Supraventricular: Originating in a pacemaker above the ventricle.

S wave: A negative wave that follows an R wave in the QRS complex.

Sympathetic nervous system: The division of the autonomic nervous system that regulates the "fight-or-flight" response, causing the heart rate and blood pressure to rise, digestion to slow, and pupils to dilate.

Syncope: Fainting spell.

Systole: The phase of the cardiac cycle in which the ventricle contracts and expels its blood.

Tachycardia: Fast heart rate, greater than 100.

T$_a$ wave: The rarely-seen wave that follows the P wave and represents repolarization of the atria.

Telemetry: A method of monitoring a patient's rhythm remotely. The patient carries a small transmitter that relays his or her cardiac rhythm to a receiver located at another location.

Thallium-201: A radioactive medication used to enable special x-ray images to be done following a stress test.

Therapeutic hypothermia: Cooling the post-cardiac arrest patient's body temperature down to 90 to 93 degrees Fahrenheit in order to decrease brain damage and improve brain function.

Thoracic: Referring to the chest cavity.

Thoracic cavity: Chest cavity.

Three-channel recorder: An EKG recorder that prints out 3 leads simultaneously.

Thrombolysis: The act of dissolving a blood clot.

Thrombolytics: Medications used to dissolve the clot causing an MI or a stroke.

Thyrotoxicosis: Also called thyroid storm. A condition in which the thyroid gland so overproduces thyroid hormones that the body's metabolic rate is accelerated to a catastrophic degree. The body temperature, heart rate, and blood pressure rise to extreme levels.

Trachea: Windpipe.

Transcutaneous: By way of the skin.

Transmembrane potential: The electrical charge at the cell membrane.

Transmural: Through the full thickness of the wall at that location.

Transvenous: By way of a vein.

Triaxial diagram: The diagram of Leads I, II, and III joined at the center or of aVR, aVL, and aVF joined at the center.

Tricuspid: Having three cusps.

Tricuspid valve: Valve that separates the right atrium and right ventricle.

Tricyclic antidepressants (TCA): A kind of medication used for the treatment of depression.

Trigeminy: Every third beat is abnormal.

Troponin: A chemical released by the heart during an MI.

Troubleshooting: Determining and correcting the cause of artifact and recording errors.

Unifocal: Coming from one location.

Unipolar: A lead consisting of only a positive pole.

Unipolar leads: Leads having only a positive pole. Unipolar leads include aVR, aVL, aVF, V1, V2, V3, V4, V5, and V6.

Unstable angina: Chest pain that is increasing in intensity and/or frequency.

Usurpation: The act of a lower pacemaker stealing control from the predominant pacemaker; results in a faster heart rate than before. Also called irritability.

U wave: A small wave sometimes seen on the EKG. It follows the T wave and reflects late repolarization.

Vagus nerve: The nerve that is part of the parasympathetic nervous system. Causes the heart rate to slow when stimulated.

Valve: A structure in the heart that prevents backflow of blood.

Vasoconstrict: To make a blood vessel's walls squeeze down, narrowing the vessel's lumen.

Vasodilate: To make the blood vessel's walls relax, thus widening the blood vessel.

Vasodilators: Medications that relax blood vessel walls.

Vector: An arrow depicting the direction of electrical current flow in the heart.

Vein: A blood vessel that transports deoxygenated blood away from the tissues.

Vena cava: The largest vein in the body; returns deoxygenated blood to the heart.

Ventricles: The lower pumping chambers of the heart.

Ventricular asystole: Another name for P wave asystole. There are P waves but no QRS complexes.

Ventricular dilatation: Stretching of the myocardial fibers from overfilling or inadequate pumping of blood from the ventricles. Results in a weakened pumping efficiency.

Ventricular ejection: The phase of systole in which the semilunar valves pop open and blood pours out of the ventricles.

Venule: A small vein that drains blood away from a capillary bed.

Index